T0259097

Neonatal Transfusion Medicine

Editors

RAVI MANGAL PATEL
AMY KEIR

CLINICS IN PERINATOLOGY

www.perinatology.theclinics.com

Consulting Editor
LUCKY JAIN

December 2023 • Volume 50 • Number 4

ELSEVIER

1600 John F. Kennedy Boulevard ● Suite 1800 ● Philadelphia, Pennsylvania, 19103-2899

http://www.theclinics.com

CLINICS IN PERINATOLOGY Volume 50, Number 4
December 2023 ISSN 0095-5108, ISBN-13: 978-0-323-96052-6

Editor: Kerry Holland
Developmental Editor: Nitesh Barthwal

Clinics in Perinatology (ISSN 0095-5108) is published quarterly by Elsevier Inc., 360 Park Avenue South, New York, NY 10010-1710. Months of issue are March, June, September, and December. Business and Editorial Offices: 1600 John F. Kennedy Blvd., Ste. 1800, Philadelphia, PA 19103-2899. Customer Service Office: 3251 Riverport Lane, Maryland Heights, MO 63043. Periodicals postage paid at New York, NY and additional mailing offices. Subscription prices are $341.00 per year (US individuals), $713.00 per year (US institutions), $387.00 per year (Canadian individuals), $872.00 per year (Canadian institutions), $461.00 per year (international individuals), $872.00 per year (international institutions), $100.00 per year (US and Canadian students), and $195.00 per year (International students). International air speed delivery is included in all Clinics subscription prices. All prices are subject to change without notice. **POSTMASTER:** Send address changes to *Clinics in Perinatology*, Elsevier Health Sciences Division, Subscription Customer Service, 3251 Riverport Lane, Maryland Heights, MO 63043. **Customer Service: Telephone: 1-800-654-2452** (U.S. and Canada); **1-314-447-8871** (outside U.S. and Canada). **Fax: 1-314-447-8029. E-mail: journalscustomerservice-usa@elsevier.com** (for print support); **journalsonlinesupport-usa@elsevier.com** (for online support).

Reprints. For copies of 100 or more, of articles in this publication, please contact the Commercial Reprints Department, Elsevier Inc., 360 Park Avenue South, New York, NY 10010-1710. Tel. 212-633-3874; Fax: 212-633-3820; E-mail: reprints@elsevier.com.

Clinics in Perinatology is also published in Spanish by McGraw-Hill Interamericana Editores S.A., P.O. Box 5-237, 06500 Mexico D.F., Mexico.

Clinics in Perinatology is covered in *MEDLINE/PubMed (Index Medicus) Current Contents, Excepta Medica,* *BIOSIS and ISI/BIOMED.*

Contributors

CONSULTING EDITOR

LUCKY JAIN, MD, MBA
Pediatrician-in-Chief, Children's Healthcare of Atlanta, George W. Brumley Jr. Professor and Chair, Emory University School of Medicine, Department of Pediatrics, Executive Director, Emory+Children's Pediatric Institute, Atlanta, Georgia, USA

EDITORS

RAVI MANGAL PATEL, MD, MSc
Professor, Department of Pediatrics, Emory University School of Medicine, Emory University, Children's Healthcare of Atlanta, Atlanta, Georgia, USA

AMY KEIR, MBBS, MPH, FRACP, PhD
Clinical Associate Professor, Adelaide Medical School, University of Adelaide and the South Australia Health and Medical Research Institute, Adelaide; Consultant Neonatologist, Women's and Children's Hospital, North Adelaide, South Australia, Australia

AUTHORS

NOUR AL-MOZAIN, MD
Consultant, Hematopathology and Transfusion Medicine, Department of Pathology and Laboratory Medicine, King Faisal Specialist Hospital and Research Centre, Clinical Assistant Professor of Hematopathology and Transfusion Medicine, Department of Pathology, College of Medicine, King Saud University, Riyadh, Saudi Arabia

CHAD C. ANDERSEN, MBBS, FRACP
Department of Perinatal Medicine, Women's and Children's Hospital, Robinson Research Institute, University of Adelaide, Adelaide, South Australia, Australia

SEAN M. BAILEY, MD
Associate Professor of Pediatrics, Division of Neonatology, Department of Pediatrics, NYU Grossman School of Medicine, Hassenfeld Children's Hospital NYU Langone, New York, New York, USA

MARIA BIANCHI, MD, PhD
Transfusion Medicine Department, Fondazione Policlinico A. Gemelli IRCCS, Roma, Italia

MICHELLE CHAPMAN, MBBS, FRACP
Neonatal Fellow, Department of Perinatal Medicine, Women's and Children's Hospital, North Adelaide, South Australia, Australia

ELIZABETH P. CROWE, MD, PhD
Assistant Professor, Department of Pathology, Johns Hopkins School of Medicine, Baltimore, Maryland, USA

GOETO DANTES, MD
General Surgeon, Department of Surgery, Emory University, Children's Healthcare of
Atlanta, Emory University School of Medicine, Emory University, Atlanta, Georgia, USA

PATRICIA DAVENPORT, MD
Neonatologist, Division of Newborn Medicine, Boston Children's Hospital, Boston,
Massachusetts, USA

SUSANNA F. FUSTOLO-GUNNINK, MD, PhD
Clinical Epidemiologist and Postdoc, Sanquin Research and Lab Services, Sanquin Blood
Supply Foundation, Almere, Amsterdam, the Netherlands

MICHAEL K. GEORGIEFF, MD
Professor, Division of Neonatology, Department of Pediatrics, University of Minnesota
Medical School, Minneapolis, Minnesota, USA

CARMEN GIANNANTONIO, MD, PhD
Neonatologist, Neonatal Intensive Care Unit, Fondazione Policlinico A. Gemelli IRCCS,
Roma, Italia

CATERINA GIOVANNA VALENTINI, MD, PhD
Hematologist, Transfusion Medicine Department, Fondazione Policlinico A. Gemelli
IRCCS, Roma, Italia

TATE GISSLEN, MD
Assistant Professor, Division of Neonatology, Department of Pediatrics, University of
Minnesota Medical School, Minneapolis, Minnesota, USA

RUCHIKA GOEL, MD, MPH
Senior Medical Director, Corporate Medical Affairs, Vitalant National Office, Scottsdale,
Arizona, USA; Associate Professor, Department of Internal Medicine and Pediatrics,
Simmons Cancer Institute at SIU School of Medicine, Springfield, Illinois, USA; Adjunct
Faculty, Department of Pathology, Johns Hopkins School of Medicine, Baltimore,
Maryland, USA

CASSANDRA D. JOSEPHSON, MD
Professor, Department of Oncology and Pediatrics, Johns Hopkins School of Medicine,
Baltimore, Maryland, USA; Director, Cancer and Blood Disorders Institute, Director,
Blood Bank and Transfusion Medicine, Department of Pathology, Johns Hopkins All
Children's Hospital, St Petersburg, Florida, USA

SARAH KEENE, MD
Assistant Professor, Emory University School of Medicine, Emory University, Department
of Neonatology, Children's Healthcare of Atlanta, Emory + Children's Pediatric Institute,
Atlanta, Georgia, USA

AMY KEIR, MBBS, MPH, FRACP, PhD
Clinical Associate Professor, Adelaide Medical School, University of Adelaide and the
South Australia Health and Medical Research Institute, Adelaide; Consultant
Neonatologist, Women's and Children's Hospital, North Adelaide, South Australia,
Australia

HARESH M. KIRPALANI
Emeritus Professor, Children's Hospital of Philadelphia, University of Pennsylvania,
Philadelphia, Pennsylvania, USA; Emeritus Professor, McMaster University, Hamilton,
Ontario, Canada

PRADEEP V. MALLY, MD
Associate Professor of Pediatrics, Division Chief, Division of Neonatology, Department of Pediatrics, NYU Grossman School of Medicine, Hassenfeld Children's Hospital NYU Langone, New York, New York, USA

PATRIZIA PAPACCI, MD
Neonatal Intensive Care Unit, Fondazione Policlinico A. Gemelli IRCCS, Università Cattolica del Sacro Cuore, Roma, Italia

RAVI MANGAL PATEL, MD, MSc
Professor, Department of Pediatrics, Emory University School of Medicine, Emory University, Children's Healthcare of Atlanta, Atlanta, Georgia, USA

RAGHAVENDRA RAO, MD
Professor, Division of Neonatology, Department of Pediatrics, University of Minnesota Medical School, Minneapolis, Minnesota, USA

ANAND SALEM, DO
Fellow in Neonatal-Perinatal Medicine, Department of Pediatrics, Emory University, Children's Healthcare of Atlanta, Atlanta, Georgia, USA

MARTHA SOLA-VISNER, MD
Division of Newborn Medicine, Boston Children's Hospital, Boston, Massachusetts, USA

ERIN SOULE-ALBRIDGE, MS
Division of Newborn Medicine, Boston Children's Hospital, Boston, Massachusetts, USA

SIMON J. STANWORTH, MA, FRCP (Paeds, UK), PhD, FRCPath
Consultant Hematologist, Professor of Hematology and Transfusion Medicine, Oxford University Hospitals NHS Trust/NHSBT/University of Oxford, Oxford, United Kingdom

MICHAEL J. STARK, PhD
Associate Professor, Department of Perinatal Medicine, Women's and Children's Hospital, Robinson Research Institute, University of Adelaide, Adelaide, South Australia, Australia

LUCIANA TEOFILI, MD, PhD
Transfusion Medicine Department, Fondazione Policlinico A. Gemelli IRCCS, Università Cattolica del Sacro Cuore, Roma, Italia

HILDE VAN DER STAAIJ, MD
Neonatologist, Neonatology Department, Willem-Alexander Children's Hospital, Leiden University Medical Center, Sanquin Research and Lab Services, Sanquin Blood Supply Foundation, Leiden, the Netherlands

GIOVANNI VENTO, MD
Neonatal Intensive Care Unit, Fondazione Policlinico A. Gemelli IRCCS, Università Cattolica del Sacro Cuore, Roma, Italia

Contents

Rapid blood loss with circulatory shock is dangerous for the preterm infant as cardiac output and oxygen-carrying capacity are simultaneously imperilled. This requires prompt restoration of circulating blood volume with emergency transfusion. *It is recommended that clinicians use both clinical and laboratory responses to guide transfusion requirements in this situation.* For preterm infants with anemia of prematurity, *it is recommended that clinicians use a restrictive algorithm from one of two recently published clinical trials.* Transfusion outside these algorithms in very preterm infants is not evidence-based and is actively discouraged.

Preterm neonates are a highly transfused patient group, with platelet transfusions being the second most transfused cellular blood component. Historically, however, evidence to inform optimal platelet transfusion practice has been limited. In pediatrics, much of the evidence has been inferred from studies in adult patients, although neonatologists have generally applied more cautious and liberal platelet transfusion thresholds to mitigate the complications of intraventricular hemorrhage. A total of three randomized controlled trials have now been published comparing different platelet transfusion strategies in neonates.

Liberal platelet transfusions are associated with increased morbidity and mortality among preterm neonates, and it is now recognized that platelets are both hemostatic and immune cells. Neonatal and adult platelets are functionally distinct, and adult platelets have the potential to be more immuno-active. Preclinical studies suggest that platelet transfusions (from adult donors) can trigger dysregulated immune responses in neonates, which might mediate the increased morbidity and mortality observed in clinical studies. More research is needed to understand how neonatal and adult platelets differ in their immune functions and the consequences of these differences in the setting of neonatal platelet transfusions.

Red blood cell transfusion is common in neonatal intensive care. Multiple trials have evaluated different thresholds for when to administer red blood cell transfusion. In contrast, there has been less focus on studies of the characteristics of red blood cells transfused into neonates. In this review, the authors summarize the emerging literature on the potential impact of the sex of blood donors on outcomes in transfused neonates using a systematic search strategy. The authors review the uncertainty generated from studies with conflicting findings and discuss considerations regarding the impact of blood donor sex and other characteristics on neonatal outcomes.

There is little formal guidance to direct neonatal blood banking practices and, as a result, practices vary widely across institutions. In this vulnerable patient population with a high transfusion burden, considerations for blood product selection include freshness, extended-storage media, pathogen inactivation, and other modifications. The authors discuss the potential unintended adverse impacts in the neonatal recipient. Concerns such as immunodeficiency, donor exposures, cytomegalovirus transmission, volume overload, transfusion-associated hyperkalemia, and passive hemolysis from ABO incompatibility have driven modifications of blood components to improve safety.

Extracorporeal Membrane Oxygenation (ECMO) is an important tool for managing critically ill neonates. Bleeding and thrombotic complications are common and significant. An understanding of ECMO physiology, its interactions with the unique neonatal hemostatic pathways, and appreciation for the distinctive risks and benefits of neonatal transfusion as it applies to ECMO are required. Currently, there is variability regarding transfusion practices, related to changing norms and a lack of high-quality literature and trials. This review provides an analysis of the neonatal ECMO transfusion literature and summarizes available best practice guidelines.

The developing brain is particularly vulnerable to extrinsic environmental events such as anemia and iron deficiency during periods of rapid development. Studies of infants with postnatal iron deficiency and iron deficiency anemia clearly demonstrated negative effects on short-term and long-term brain development and function. Randomized interventional trials studied erythropoiesis-stimulating agents and hemoglobin-based red blood cell transfusion thresholds to determine how they affect preterm infant neurodevelopment. Studies of red blood cell transfusion components are limited in preterm neonates. A biomarker strategy measuring brain iron status and health in the preanemic period is desirable to evaluate treatment options and brain response.

Patient blood management (PBM) is an evidence-based care package to improve patient outcomes by optimizing a patient's blood, minimizing blood loss, and the effective management and, when appropriate, the tolerance of anemia. It is relatively well-developed in adult medicine and remains in its infancy in neonatology. This review explores why evidence-based guidelines are insufficient, discusses the variations in neonatal transfusion practice and why this matters, and provides the key updates in neonatal transfusion practice. The authors give examples of a successful neonatal PBM program and single-center projects.

Repeated red blood cell (RBC) transfusions in preterm neonates cause the progressive displacement of fetal hemoglobin (HbF) by adult hemoglobin. The ensuing increase of oxygen delivery may result at the cellular level in a dangerous condition of hyperoxia, explaining the association between low-HbF levels and retinopathy of prematurity or bronchopulmonary dysplasia. Transfusing preterm neonates with RBC concentrates obtained from allogeneic umbilical blood is a strategy to increase hemoglobin concentration without depleting the physiologic HbF reservoir. This review summarizes the mechanisms underlying a plausible beneficial impact of this strategy and reports clinical experience gathered so far in this field.

This review is a summary of available evidence regarding the use of near-infrared spectroscopy (NIRS) to help better guide and understand the effects of red blood cell (RBC) transfusion in neonatal patients. We review recent literature demonstrating the changes that take place in regional tissue oxygen saturation (rSO_2) resulting from RBC transfusion. We also discuss in detail if any correlation exists between rSO_2 and hemoglobin values in neonates. Finally, we review studies that have evaluated the use of NIRS as a transfusion guide during neonatal intensive care.

PROGRAM OBJECTIVE
The goal of *Clinics in Perinatology* is to keep practicing perinatologists, neonatologists, obstetricians, practicing physicians and residents up to date with current clinical practice in perinatology by providing timely articles reviewing the state of the art in patient care.

TARGET AUDIENCE
Perinatologists, neonatologists, obstetricians, practicing physicians, residents and healthcare professionals who provide patient care utilizing findings from *Clinics in Perinatology*.

LEARNING OBJECTIVES
Upon completion of this activity, participants will be able to:
1. Recognize changes in current practice likely to improve outcomes in neonatal transfusions.
2. Discuss considerations for blood product selection concerning the neonatal population.
3. Review evidence-based guidelines to improve neonatal patient blood management.

ACCREDITATION
The Elsevier Office of Continuing Medical Education (EOCME) is accredited by the Accreditation Council for Continuing Medical Education (ACCME) to provide continuing medical education for physicians.

The EOCME designates this journal-based CME activity for a maximum of 10 *AMA PRA Category 1 Credit*(s)™. Physicians should claim only the credit commensurate with the extent of their participation in the activity.

All other health care professionals requesting continuing education credit for this enduring material will be issued a certificate of participation.

DISCLOSURE OF CONFLICTS OF INTEREST
The EOCME assesses conflict of interest with its instructors, faculty, planners, and other individuals who are in a position to control the content of CME activities. All relevant conflicts of interest that are identified are thoroughly vetted by EOCME for fair balance, scientific objectivity, and patient care recommendations. EOCME is committed to providing its learners with CME activities that promote improvements or quality in healthcare and not a specific proprietary business or a commercial interest.

The planning committee, staff, authors, and editors listed below have identified no financial relationships or relationships to products or devices they or their spouse/life partner have with commercial interest related to the content of this CME activity:
Nour Al Mozain, MD; Chad C. Andersen, MBBS, FRACP; Maria Bianchi, MD, PhD; Michelle Chapman, MBBS, FRACP; Elizabeth P. Crowe, MD, PhD; Goeto Dantes, MD; Patricia Davenport, MD; Susanna F. Fustolo-Gunnink, MD, PhD; Michael K. Georgieff, MD; Carmen Giannantonio, MD, PhD; Tate Gisslen, MD; Sarah Keene, MD; Amy K. Keir, MBBS, MPH, FRACP, PhD; Haresh M. Kirpalani, MD, MSc; Michelle Littlejohn; Pradeep V. Mally, MD; Patrizia Papacci, MD; Raghavendra Rao, MD; Anand Salem, DO; Martha Sola-Visner, MD; Erin Soule-Albridge, MS; Simon J. Stanworth, MA, FRCP (Paeds, UK), PhD, FRCPath; Michael J. Stark, PhD; Jeyanthi Surendrakumar; Luciana Teofili, MD, PhD; Caterina Giovanna Valentini, MD, PhD; Hilde van der Staaij, MD; Giovanni Vento, MD

The planning committee, staff, authors, and editors listed below have identified financial relationships or relationships to products or devices they or their spouse/life partner have with commercial interest related to the content of this CME activity:
Sean M. Bailey, MD: Speaker: Medtronic

Ruchika Goel, MD, MPH: Advisor: Rigel Pharmaceuticals

Cassandra D. Josephson, MD: Researcher: Medtronic

Ravi M. Patel, MD, MSc: Consultant/Advisor: Noveome

UNAPPROVED/OFF-LABEL USE DISCLOSURE
The EOCME requires CME faculty to disclose to the participants:
1. When products or procedures being discussed are off-label, unlabelled, experimental, and/or investigational (not US Food and Drug Administration [FDA] approved); and
2. Any limitations on the information presented, such as data that are preliminary or that represent ongoing research, interim analyses, and/or unsupported opinions. Faculty may discuss information about pharmaceutical agents that is outside of FDA-approved labelling. This information is intended solely for CME

and is not intended to promote off-label use of these medications. If you have any questions, contact the medical affairs department of the manufacturer for the most recent prescribing information.

TO ENROLL
To enroll in the *Clinics in Perinatology* Continuing Medical Education program, call customer service at 1-800-654-2452 or sign up online at http://www.theclinics.com/home/cme. The CME program is available to subscribers for an additional annual fee of USD 254.00.

METHOD OF PARTICIPATION
In order to claim credit, participants must complete the following:
1. Complete enrolment as indicated above.
2. Read the activity.
3. Complete the CME Test and Evaluation. Participants must achieve a score of 70% on the test. All CME Tests and Evaluations must be completed online.

CME INQUIRIES/SPECIAL NEEDS
For all CME inquiries or special needs, please contact elsevierCME@elsevier.com.

CLINICS IN PERINATOLOGY

SERIES OF RELATED INTEREST

Obstetrics and Gynecology Clinics of North America
https://www.obgyn.theclinics.com

THE CLINICS ARE AVAILABLE ONLINE!
Access your subscription at:
www.theclinics.com

Foreword
The Future of Transfusion Medicine .

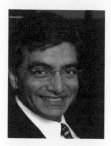

Lucky Jain, MD, MBA
Consulting Editor

Much progress has been made in transfusion medicine since the turn of the nineteenth century when the discovery of blood group antigens made a significant dent in mismatched transfusions and ushered in a new era of science and innovation. Better collection and preservation of blood products, accompanied by accurate testing, tracking, and documentation of essential data, have all essentially reduced transfusion-related errors to a bare minimum. Blood banks now rely on advanced automations and algorithms to manage a wide range of blood products rather than relying on manual records and human judgment.

So where do we go from here? One of the biggest achievements in recent years is the acceptance of transfusion medicine as a unique discipline within medicine with specific training requirements and certifications. Availability of trained professionals allowed for precision in transfusion decisions, resulting in better outcomes and conservation of blood products. It also allowed for rigorous tracking of transfusion safety through a "vein-to-vein" digital footprint, including digital labeling of all blood products with technologies such as Radio Frequency Identification (RFID) (**Fig. 1**).[1,2] There is also the hope that artificial intelligence, machine learning, and deep learning approaches will bring efficiencies and accuracy to all aspects of transfusion medicine. Electronic order sets and transfusion protocols will not only reduce human error but also facilitate accumulation of data that can guide further improvements.

Use of blood products in neonates and young infants continues to evolve with many studies addressing threshold levels for transfusion for red blood cells and platelets. Modern techniques, such as transfusion medicine, genome-wide genotyping array, and metabolomics, will help in refining practices.[3,4] Approaches under investigation

Clin Perinatol 50 (2023) xv–xvii
https://doi.org/10.1016/j.clp.2023.09.003
0095-5108/23/© 2023 Published by Elsevier Inc.

perinatology.theclinics.com

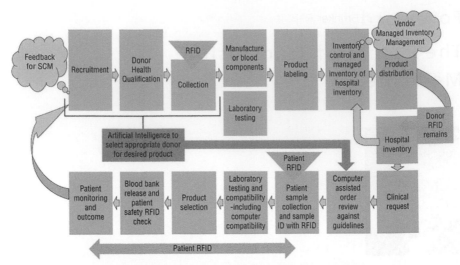

Fig. 1. Flow of a potential digital footprint of the integration of RFID into the vein-to-vein transfusion chain.[1,2] (With permission from Smit Sibinga CTh. Transfusion medicine: From ABO to AI (artificial intelligence). In Linwood SI., editor Digital Health. Brisbane (AU): Exon Publications. Online first 2022. Feb 22.)

include next-generation sequencing for exome sequencing, whole-genome sequencing, or polymerase chain reaction–based targeted next-generation sequencing methods.[3]

It has been many years since the publication of an entire issue of the *Clinics in Perinatology* devoted to transfusion medicine. In this current issue, Drs Patel and Keir have expanded the scope and purpose of transfusion medicine by assembling an extraordinary list of experts in the field. They are all to be congratulated for a truly state-of-the-art offering on this subject. As always, I am grateful to the authors for their valuable contributions and to my publishing partners at Elsevier (Kerry Holland and Nitesh Barthwal) for their help in bringing this valuable resource to you.

Lucky Jain, MD, MBA
Department of Pediatrics
Emory University School of Medicine
Children's Healthcare of Atlanta
2015 Uppergate Drive NE
Atlanta, GA 30322, USA

E-mail address:
ljain@emory.edu

REFERENCES

1. Smit Sibinga CTh. Transfusion medicine: from ABO to AI (artificial intelligence). In: Linwood SI, editor. Digital health. Brisbane (AU): Exon Publications; 2022.

2. Holmberg J. The digital footprint in transfusion medicine and the potential for vein-to-vein management, 2018, Medical Laboratory Observer, Available at: http://www.mlo-online.com/information-technology/automation/article/13017030/the-digital-footprint-in-transfusion-medicine-and-the-potential-for-veintovein-management. Accessed September 17, 2023.

3. Montemayor C, Brunker PAR, Keller M. Banking with precision: transfusion medicine as a potential universal application in clinical genomics. Curr Opin Hematol 2019;26(6):480–7. https://doi.org/10.1097/MOH.0000000000000536.
4. Nemkov T, Hansen KC, Dumont LJ, et al. Metabolomics in transfusion medicine. Transfusion 2016;56(4):980–93. https://doi.org/10.1111/trf.13442.

Preface

Understanding the WHEN, WHAT, and WHY of Neonatal Transfusion Medicine

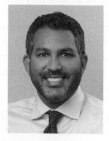 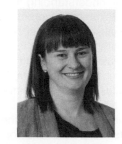

Ravi Mangal Patel, MD, MSc   Amy Keir, MBBS, MPH, PhD
Editors

What an exciting time in neonatal transfusion medicine! It has been over 8 years since the last issue of *Clinics in Perinatology* on neonatal hematology and transfusion medicine was published.[1] Much has happened in the intervening years. We are honored to serve as Guest Editors of this exciting issue on Neonatal Transfusion Medicine.

We've learned much about red blood cell transfusion thresholds in extremely preterm neonates through two recent trials: TOP[2] and ETTNO.[3] These important trials have provided critical evidence on *when* to transfuse extremely preterm neonates and are discussed in detail in the article, "Thresholds for Red Blood Cell Transfusion in Preterm Infants: Evidence to Practice," by Andersen and colleagues. However, tolerating anemia with more restrictive practices than studied may also have consequences, and the article, "Anemia, Iron Supplementation, and the Brain," by Gisslen and colleagues discusses some considerations about the effects of anemia and iron supplementation on the brain. Clinical evidence alone may not be sufficient to change practice[4]; the article, "Patient Blood Management in Neonates," by Chapman and Keir discusses the role of patient blood management in translating research findings into routine neonatal care to improve blood utilization. Looking ahead to improving the precision of guiding red blood cell transfusion beyond a hemoglobin measurement and *why* we transfuse neonates, the article, "Near-Infrared Spectroscopy to Guide and Understand Effects of Red Blood Cell Transfusion," by Bailey and Mally explores the use of near-infrared spectroscopy to identify the need for and understand the effects of red blood cell transfusion. Our field needs more evidence on transfusion in populations of term infants. One such population is neonates receiving extracorporeal membrane oxygenation (ECMO), among the highest utilizers of blood products, which is

Clin Perinatol 50 (2023) xix–xxi
https://doi.org/10.1016/j.clp.2023.09.002
0095-5108/23/© 2023 Published by Elsevier Inc.

reviewed in "Transfusion in Neonatal Extracorporeal Membrane Oxygenation: A Best Practice Review" by Dantes and Keene.

For platelet transfusion, a big jolt to neonatal transfusion medicine came with the findings of the PlaNeT-2 trial.[5] This trial supports lower platelet transfusion thresholds, often much lower than those being used in routine practice.[6] "Prophylactic Platelet Transfusions: Why Less Is More" by van der Staaij and colleagues discusses this trial in detail, and "Hemostatic and Immunologic Effects of Platelet Transfusions in Neonates" by Davenport and colleagues provides mechanistic insights on the biological effects of platelet transfusions.

Beyond just *when* to transfuse is understanding the impact of *what* is being transfused. The articles "Blood Donor Sex and Outcomes in Transfused Infants" by Salem and Patel and "Neonatal Blood Banking Practices" by Crowe and colleagues discuss the potential importance of the characteristics of the blood products and their donors that are used for neonatal transfusion. We round out this series with the article, "Allogenic Cord Blood Transfusion in Preterm Infants" by Teofili and colleagues, which reviews allogenic cord blood transfusion in preterm infants. This could be a pioneering new strategy to change *what* we transfuse.[7]

We would like to express our sincere gratitude to the authors of this issue, who are respected colleagues and experts in the field. We hope you share our excitement of the recent progress in neonatal transfusion medicine that is summarized in this issue.

DISCLOSURES

Dr R.M. Patel receives funding from the National Institutes of Health and unrestricted equipment support from Medtronic. Dr A. Keir receives funding from the Australian National Health and Medical Research Council (NHMRC) (APP1161379).

Ravi Mangal Patel, MD, MSc
Emory University School of Medicine and
Children's Healthcare of Atlanta
2015 Uppergate Drive NE
Atlanta, GA 30322, USA

Amy Keir, MBBS, MPH, PhD
South Australia Health and
Medical Research Institute
72 King William Road
North Adelaide, SA 5006, Australia

E-mail addresses:
rmpatel@emory.edu (R.M. Patel)
amy.keir@adelaide.edu.au (A. Keir)

REFERENCES

1. Christensen RD, Juul SE, Del Vecchio A. The expanding evidence base to guide neonatal hematology and transfusion medicine practice. Preface. Clin Perinatol 2015;42(3):xix–xxx. https://doi.org/10.1016/j.clp.2015.05.002.

2. Kirpalani H, Bell EF, Hintz SR, et al. Higher or Lower Hemoglobin Transfusion Thresholds for Preterm Infants. N Engl J Med 2020;383(27):2639–51.

3. Franz AR, Engel C, Bassler D, et al. Effects of liberal vs restrictive transfusion thresholds on survival and neurocognitive outcomes in extremely low-birth-weight

infants: the ETTNO randomized clinical trial. JAMA 2020;324(6):560–70. https://doi.org/10.1001/jama.2020.10690.

4. Keir A, Grace E, Stanworth S. Closing the evidence to practice gap in neonatal transfusion medicine. Semin Fetal Neonatal Med 2021;26(1):101197. https://doi.org/10.1016/j.siny.2021.101197.

5. Curley A, Stanworth SJ, Willoughby K, et al. Randomized Trial of Platelet-Transfusion Thresholds in Neonates. N Engl J Med 2019;380(3):242–51.

6. Patel RM, Hendrickson JE, Nellis ME, et al. Variation in neonatal transfusion practice. J Pediatr 2021;235:92–9.e4. https://doi.org/10.1016/j.jpeds.2021.04.002.

7. Teofili L, Papacci P, Orlando N, et al. BORN study: a multicenter randomized trial investigating cord blood red blood cell transfusions to reduce the severity of retinopathy of prematurity in extremely low gestational age neonates. Trials 2022; 23(1):1010.

Thresholds for Red Blood Cell Transfusion in Preterm Infants: Evidence to Practice

Chad C. Andersen, MBBS, FRACP[a],*, Michael J. Stark[a],
Haresh M. Kirpalani[b,c]

KEYWORDS

• Newborn • Infant • Hemoglobin • Blood • Transfusion • Oxygen

KEY POINTS

- Rapid blood loss with circulatory shock imperils oxygen handling in the preterm infant.
- Anemic shock requires prompt restoration of circulating blood volume with emergency transfusion.
- Infants with anemia of prematurity should be transfused according to a published restrictive hemoglobin threshold algorithm.
- Transfusion outside these algorithms in very preterm infants is not evidence-based.

PREAMBLE

... that I do not think I know what I do not know...

[Plato's Apology to Socrates]

Allogeneic red blood cell (RBC) transfusion remains one of the most frequent interventions in very preterm infants.[1] For decades, the discipline of neonatal medicine has sought a one-rule-for-all approach for this common therapy. However, this idea is fundamentally flawed as no two infants have the same oxygen physiology, similar concurrent morbidities, or comparable environmental conditions.[2,3] Despite these differences being apparent to the clinician, the approach to transfusion has remained embedded in an inflexible, center-specific framework.

---

[a] Department of Perinatal Medicine, Women's and Children's Hospital and Robinson Research Institute, University of Adelaide, South Australia; [b] Children's Hospital of Philadelphia at University Pennsylvania, Philadelphia, USA; [c] McMaster University, Hamilton, Ontario, Canada
* Corresponding author. Department of Perinatal Medicine, Women's and Children's Hospital, Level 1, Queen Victoria Building, 72 King William Road, North Adelaide, South Australia 5006.
E-mail address: chad.andersen@sa.gov.au

Clin Perinatol 50 (2023) 763–774
https://doi.org/10.1016/j.clp.2023.07.001
0095-5108/23/Crown Copyright © 2023 Published by Elsevier Inc. All rights reserved.
perinatology.theclinics.com

Why Does This Approach Require Redefining?

Until recently, RBC transfusion was erroneously regarded as biologically inert.[4–6] In addition, the critical threshold for anemic hypoxia, when end-organ hypoxemia commences, varies in each organ within each infant. Although this makes the application of a physiologic transfusion algorithm almost impossible in the clinical setting, we suggest that attempts to individualize transfusion requirements in preterm infants remain a priority. Although we acknowledge that this requires further research with a particular focus given to the link between the clinical situation and contemporaneous physiology.

INTRODUCTION

RBC transfusion is an allograft, that is, a biologically active tissue that is transplanted from one person—a donor, to another—the recipient. The only indisputable reason to justify transfusion is to avoid end-organ injury from hyperbilirubinemia (exchange transfusion) or hypoxemia,[7] although these are both difficult to define in a preterm infant. With respect to hypoxemia, not only does the form of hypoxemia alter the threshold at which injury commences but also the type of hemoglobin (Hb) being transfused may also be critical.[8]

However, blood has been used for several clinical reasons, many of which are not evidence-based.[9–17] Historically, indications include low hemoglobin (Hb) or hematocrit (Hct) value,[18] poor weight gain,[9] apnea of prematurity,[19,20] "suboptimal oxygenation" (exchange transfusion of adult RBCs),[21] retinopathy of prematurity,[22] bronchopulmonary dysplasia,[23] necrotizing enterocolitis[24] and hyperbilirubinemia (at least before the widespread use of phototherapy). The transfusion product has also changed from whole blood in glass vials to concentrated (higher hematocrit), leukodepleted RBCs suspended in a glucose and phosphate solution and supplied as multipacks from a single donor.[25–28] These practice changes have lowered donor exposure and therefore the risk of transfusion-acquired viral infection. Despite the move away from transfusion of whole blood and particularly with prestorage leukoreduction, some centers irradiate allogeneic blood for all transfusions due to the small risk of graft versus host disease (GVHD), whereas others do only irradiate RBCs to be used in the context of fetal or exchange transfusion.[29,30]

Center and individual clinician-based variation in practice and differences in the transfusion product challenges the evidence-based decision-making.[31,32] Further complexity arises from bundling historical with contemporary literature. This is particularly relevant to clinical outcomes in preterm babies, with many greatly affected by other advances in neonatal medicine, such as the administration of antenatal steroids.[33] Moreover, although the neurodevelopmental outcome of surviving preterm babies is a particular focus for the neonatal clinician, the effects of anemia on longer term outcomes other than mortality are not explicitly reported in transfusion trials in adult populations.

CURRENT EVIDENCE IN OTHER POPULATIONS

The American Association of Blood Banks recommends a restrictive practice of RBC transfusion in sick, hospitalized adults but allows consideration for specific clinical situations. This advice is derived from a systematic review of several large, randomized trials showing no difference in 30-day mortality between adults transfused according to a restrictive or liberal transfusion practice ($n = 12587$ overall, relative risk [RR] 0.97 [CI 0.81, 1.16]).[34] For paediatric patients, including those who are critically ill, the

Australian National Blood Authority's Patient Blood Management Guidelines, Module 6—Neonatal and Pediatrics, also recommends the use of a restrictive RBC transfusion threshold.[35] However, the level of evidence for this recommendation was low (GRADE C), highlighting the need for care to be taken in its application.[34]

WHEN SHOULD THE PRETERM INFANT BE TRANSFUSED?

This is a deceptively simple question that is complex to answer. This is partly due to the wide range of indications for transfusion in the neonatal population. Furthermore, the clinical and physiologic responses to this common intervention are influenced by the primary reason for transfusion combined with the effect of transfusion exposure itself.[36]

Brief Physiology

RBC transfusion increases Hb concentration and may reduce the short and possible long-term consequences of anemic hypoxia. However, this presumes that tissue oxygen delivery improves with the correction of anemia.[37] Our own work shows that transfusion reduces cerebral oxygen extraction, consistent with the likely physiology though it is, at present, unable to resolve the requirement for transfusion.[38]

A low circulating RBC count is usually determined by measuring Hb or Hct. However, although Hb is important for oxygen uptake and delivery, no single value defines anemic hypoxia in all babies, that is, there is no universal threshold for anemic hypoxia as oxygen physiology is dynamic in the individual.[39] This means that the interpretation of each Hb value depends on the oxygen physiology *at the time* of measurement. As a result, any rule will be imperfect as oxygen consumption and delivery is in constant flux. This concept refutes a *one-rule-for-all* approach in clinical practice.

The primary function of hemoglobin is to carry oxygen: How does this process work?

Oxygen diffuses down a concentration gradient from the alveolar space to the mitochondrion.[40] This carefully preserved process has many checks and balances, including alveolar ventilation, hemoglobin—oxygen binding, blood flow, and passive diffusion. Following diffusion into the plasma, oxygen rapidly moves across the RBC membrane and into the cytoplasm before binding to Hb.

Systemic blood flow, Hb concentration, and the oxygen saturation of Hb are the three primary determinants of systemic oxygen delivery.[40] However, although the diffusion distance and the oxygen gradient between blood and the cell are essential in the microvasculature,[41] they are of minor importance overall.

Oxygen consumption drives oxygen kinetics and is in constant flux, requiring a system-wide buffering capacity to safeguard aerobic metabolism. Compensation for alterations in oxygen consumption or oxygen delivery, or both, requires a dynamic and responsive process. Variable extraction of oxygen from oxyhemoglobin provides this capability.[42] However, when compensation is extinguished, oxygen consumption becomes restricted by oxygen delivery. At this point, anaerobic metabolism begins with the accumulation of lactic acid in the body (*anaerobic debt*).[43] A hypothetical value, known as the *critical threshold*, defines that point of restricted oxygen metabolism. Although this is conceptually significant, it varies according to the mechanism of hypoxia and, as such, it is very difficult to define in preterm infants.[37,44,45]

Last, the molecular structure of Hb changes in late gestation and throughout the first year of life. This structural change, from fetal (HbF) to adult hemoglobin (HbA), alters the affinity of Hb for oxygen. The higher affinity of HbF (lower $p50$) facilitates oxygen diffusion from the maternal–placental interface.[8]

Packed red blood cells for transfusion

Following collection, whole blood is separated into components with the RBC concentrate typically resuspended in high-concentration glucose with inorganic phosphate and stored at 1 and 6°C. This product degrades over time as RBC metabolism continues, leading to a *storage lesion* with oxidative damage, cell lysis with the liberation of iron, depletion of 2,3 diphosphoglycerate (2,3 DPG) and elevation of lactate.[46] This worsens with the length of storage. However, trials in adults, children, infants, and neonates show no difference in clinical outcomes with fresh compared with moderately aged blood (adults n = 4686, RR1.04 [95%CI 0.95, 1.15], children, infants, and neonates n = 829, RR 1.04 [95%CI 0.94, 1.14]).[34,47,48]

Last, irradiating RBC products before transfusion is still recommended in several jurisdictions primarily to reduce the risk of GVHD.[49] However, gamma irradiation damages the blood product, liberates potassium, and reduces the shelf life,[50] although the clinical implication of this treatment is unclear.[51,52]

FROM CONCEPT TO PRACTICE: WHEN SHOULD THE PRETERM BABY BE TRANSFUSED?

There are two broad clinical scenarios in which RBC transfusion is typically used.

Scenario 1

A baby is delivered following an antepartum hemorrhage in the setting of a vasa praevia. At birth, the baby has evidence of circulatory (anemic) shock, tachycardia, hypotension, a low Hb value, and elevated lactate.

Summary

This baby has acute anemic shock (hypovolemic anemia). This might similarly happen during a surgical procedure with rapid blood loss, for example.

Cardiac output (a combination of stroke volume and heart rate) is imperilled in this scenario, as the heart requires a preload "filling" condition to maintain stroke volume. Transfusion of RBCs will rapidly restore both circulating blood volume and oxygen-carrying capacity. The threshold for transfusion is hard to quantify in this situation as it depends on the volume and speed of blood loss. Key indicators for urgent RBC transfusion include clinical signs such as pallor, tachycardia, hypotension, and deteriorating conscious state. Laboratory values are also important, including falling Hbmore often a later finding, abnormal coagulation profile with acidosis, and increasing lactate. Transfusion will restore preload condition, thereby improving stroke volume and increasing oxygen-carrying capacity. Although there are no randomized trials in preterm infants to guide clinical practice in this setting, there is other supportive information from animal models.[53]

Recommendation

Babies with anemic shock require prompt administration of RBCs. However, there is no established method to determine the replacement volume. Instead, it is recommended that the bedside clinician infuse RBCs in aliquots of 10 mLs/kg, measuring the effect of each volume on hemodynamic (heart rate and blood pressure) and laboratory (Hb value, lactate) responses. This might require transfusion volumes of different sizes delivered over variable time intervals.

Scenario 2

A very low birth weight baby, delivered at 25 weeks, who is now 3 weeks of age, has a Hb value of 80 g/dL. The baby requires respiratory *support* and a small amount of supplemental oxygen. She has normal blood pressure and heart rate and is otherwise well.

Summary

This baby likely has normovolemic anemia, typically the result of anemia of prematurity. For the purpose of clinical assessment, normovolemia can be defined as normotension without tachycardia, normal urine volume, and absence of lactic acidosis.

Of both scenarios, this is the most common particularly in the preterm baby, as a result of anemia of prematurity.[54,55] Large phlebotomy losses coupled with a poorly responsive bone marrow often result in normovolemic anemia in the preterm baby.[55] Whereas this pattern is similar to that described in the normal term baby, in the preterm infant, the fall in Hb is earlier, as a result of the phlebotomy losses associated with acuity, more gradual and more profound. Typically, babies are "topped up" or transfused according to a Hb or hematocrit value derived from clinical experience. Although a threshold implies a response around a particular value, this may not be the same in each infant. The threshold suggests that each Hb value is dichotomous, yet, in truth, Hb is a continuous variable.

Six randomized trials evaluate an approach to transfusion using Hb or Hct thresholds.[56–62] In each trial, infants were assigned to one algorithm, characteristically described as liberal or an alternate, typically described as restrictive. The earlier transfusion trials are less relevant today partly because of the lower use of antenatal steroids. Further, there is a potential greater validity of larger trials over smaller ones, though this is debated.[63,64] Nonetheless, two recent trials dominate the pooled analysis.[65] These trials are structured differently from earlier studies. They include a primary composite outcome of death or neurodevelopmental impairment up to 24 months post-conceptual age. In addition, they also report important secondary outcomes, including but not limited to necrotizing enterocolitis. Both trials are similarly designed, with comparable populations, yet have subtle but potentially significant differences in the approach to transfusion. They are also the only trials providing data of relevance for longer term neurosensory outcomes with no meaningful attrition bias.

Both trials used Hb or hematocrit thresholds for transfusion varying by chronologic age and illness acuity, reflecting concern that the risk of short and long-term morbidity is highest in the first weeks of life. Although fixed Hb thresholds determine transfusion, additional transfusions were permitted in situations such as critical illness or surgery, reflecting contemporaneous practice. Importantly, the trials were analyzed by intention-to-treat and had very high rates of neurodevelopmental follow-up, though at slightly different ages and with different psychometric tests.

The *Effects of Transfusion Thresholds on Outcomes of Extremely Low-Birth-Weight Infant* (ETTNO) trial enrolled infants (*n* = 1013), between 400 and 999 grams AND less than 30 completed weeks gestation at birth, in 36 centers, before 72 hours of age.[58] The trial was stratified by weight and center. In addition, 516 infants were exposed to a center-specific higher saturation target in comparison to 407 infants who were managed with a center-specific lower saturation target. In 34 of 36 centers, measurement was based on either venous or arterial Hct. In comparison to the Transfusion in Preterms (TOP) trial, infants had a higher Hb at randomization, likely reflecting a systematic difference, such as more widespread delayed cord clamping or transfusion before study enrolment. A fixed transfusion volume of 20 mLs/kg was given, and 64% received irradiated blood. The study was powered to detect a 10% absolute risk reduction of a primary composite outcome of death and neurodevelopmental disability at 24 months post-conceptual age. Seven hundred sixty-five infants (of 1013 total) were assessed with the Bayley Scales of Infant Development II. The sample

Table 1
Outcomes from the Effects of Transfusion Thresholds on Outcomes of Extremely Low-Birth-Weight Infant and Transfusion in Preterms trials according to the allocated thresholds for transfusion

| | Clinical Trial | | | | Analysis of Restrictive Versus Liberal |
| | Restrictive | | Liberal | | |
Outcome	ETTNO	TOP	ETTNO	TOP	
Hb (g/dL) at trial entry	15.5 ± (2.4)	13.7 ± 2.6	15.1 ± (2.3)	13.8 ± 2.6	RD −0.13 (−0.15, −0.1)
Transfused more than once (%)	311/521 (59)	804/913 (88)	391/492 (79)	885/911 (97)	
Transfusion per infant (Mean [SD])	2 (2.6) (n = 521)	4.4 (4) (n = 912)	2.9 (2.5) (n = 492)	6.2 (4.3) (n = 911)	MD −1.27 (−1.51, −1.02)
Death (primary hospital discharge) (%)	38/515 (7.4)	125/913 (13.6)	36/488 (7.4)	127/911 (13.9)	RR 0.99 (0.8, 1.21)
Neurosensory impairment (%)	148/430 (34)	287/712 (40)	154/410 (38)	277/699 (40)	RR 0.99 (0.89, 1.09)
Death or neurodevelopmental impairment (%)	205/478 (43)	422/847 (50.1)	200/450 (44)	423/845 (50)	RR 1.02 (0.94, 1.1)
Retinopathy of prematurity (ROP) (Grade 3 or greater) (%)	64/492 (13)	137/797 (17)	175/472 (6)	157/797 (20)	RR 0.85 (0.72, 1.02)
Necrotizing enterocolitis (NEC) Bell stage 2 or greater (%)	32/518 (6)	95/906 (11)	26/492 (5)	91/907 (10)	RR 0.94 (0.74, 1.19)
Bronchopulmonary dysplasia (BPD) (Supplemental O_2 or respiratory support at 36 wk post menstrual age [PMA]) (%)	126/485 (26)	453/805 (56)	130/458 (28)	469/795 (59)	RR 0.95 (0.87, 1.02)

Table 2
Cognitive outcomes, separated by psychometric test, from the Effects of Transfusion Thresholds on Outcomes of Extremely Low-Birth-Weight Infant and Transfusion in Preterms trials according to the allocated thresholds for transfusion

Outcome		Restrictive	Liberal	Risk Ratio
Cognitive delay < 70	Bayley II or physician Bayley III	62/387 (14.4%) 96/712 (13.5%)	71/378 (17.3) 88/695 (12.7%)	1.03 (0.84, 1.26)
Cognitive delay <85	Bayley II Bayley III	139/387 (32%) 270/712 (38%)	143/378 (34.8%) 269/695 (38.7%)	1.02 (0.91, 1.13)

size was based on the effect size of the premature infants in need of transfusion trial.[57] There was no interaction between the saturation target (non-randomized) and the allocated hematocrit algorithm.

The TOP trial enrolled infants ($n = 1824$) who were greater than 22 weeks but less than 28 completed weeks gestation AND less than 1000 grams AND less than 48 hours of age in 19 centers. Infants were excluded if they received erythropoietin or a transfusion after 6 hours of life or.[56] Irradiated blood was used in all infants. Enrolled infants were randomly allocated to either a liberal or restrictive transfusion threshold based on the hemoglobin value, with thresholds varying according to chronologic age and illness severity (**Tables 1–3**). A fixed volume of 15 mLs/kg was used. The study was powered to detect a 7% absolute difference in the primary outcome between trial groups, and like the ETTNO trial, a primary cluster outcome of death and neurodevelopmental disability at later follow-up was used. Infants were assessed using the Bayley Scales of Infant Development III at 22 to 26 months post-conceptual age.

Table 3
Transfusion thresholds, converted to hemoglobin values, from the Effects of Transfusion Thresholds on Outcomes of Extremely Low-Birth-Weight Infant and Transfusion in Preterms trials

	FTTNO		TOP	
Transfusion volume (mLs/kg)	20		15	
	Critical health state[a]		Respiratory support[b]	
	Restrictive	Liberal	Restrictive	Liberal
Week 1	116	139	110	130
Week 2	102	126	100	125
Week 3	93	116	85	110
	Noncritical health state		No respiratory support	
	Restrictive	Liberal	Restrictive	Liberal
Week 1	95	119	100	120
Week 2	82	105	85	110
Week 3	71	95	70	100

[a] Critical health state was defined as an infant having at least one of the following criteria: invasive mechanical ventilation, continuous positive airway pressure with a fraction of inspired oxygen >0.25 for >12 hours per 24 hours, treatment for patent ductus arteriosus, acute sepsis, or necrotizing enterocolitis with circulatory failure requiring inotropic/vasopressor support, >6 nurse-documented apneas requiring intervention per 24 hours, or >4 intermittent hypoxemic episodes with pulse oximetry oxygen saturation.
[b] Respiratory support was defined as mechanical ventilation, continuous positive airway pressure, a fraction of inspired oxygen (FiO_2) greater than 0.35, or delivery of oxygen or room air by nasal cannula at a flow of 1 L per minute or more.

A potential bias in both trials was the relatively high rates of noncompliant transfusion, particularly in infants allocated to the restrictive transfusion algorithms [liberal 5% (ETTNO) and 0.8% (TOP) compared with restrictive 15% (ETTNO) and 7.4% (TOP)]. This reflects the complex clinical environment in this population and the pragmatic nature of both trials.

These trials, separately and together ($n = 2837$ infants from 55 centers), show no difference in the outcome of death or neurosensory impairment in very preterm babies transfused according to a liberal OR restrictive Hb threshold value (see **Tables 1** and **2**). However, infants allocated to the restrictive threshold received fewer transfusions overall, suggesting that a restrictive approach reduces transfusion exposure without worsening important outcomes.

Recommendation

Very preterm infants, who are born less than 30 weeks gestational age, should be transfused according to the restrictive arm of either the ETTNO or TOP trials (see **Table 3**) with the volume of transfusion in keeping with the trial algorithm used. The use of thresholds outside those used in the trials is strongly discouraged.

Last, there is very little evidence to guide transfusion practice in mature newborns.

SUMMARY

The prospect of improving *oxygenation*, in an anemic recipient, with a RBC transfusion is compelling. However, the effect of allogeneic adult red cell transfusion on an immature recipient is complex. Red cell transfusion may improve the preload condition of the heart, favorably altering oxygen-carrying capacity while modifying the Hb—oxygen affinity to assist tissue unloading. Despite these potential advantageous effects, concerns remain about transfusion-related harm. Balancing these competing effects is difficult for the clinician.

Blood transfusion is typically considered in two scenarios defined by circulating blood volume. Rapid blood loss with circulatory shock is dangerous for the preterm infant as both cardiac output and oxygen-carrying capacity are simultaneously imperilled. This clinical situation requires prompt restoration of circulating blood volume with RBCs. The quantity and speed of administration will vary in each clinical situation. *It is recommended that clinicians use both clinical and laboratory responses to guide transfusion requirements.* For preterm infants with anemia of prematurity, *it is recommended that clinicians use one of the restrictive hemoglobin or hematocrit threshold algorithms from two large clinical trials* as they show no short or longer term disadvantage to transfusion at restrictive thresholds yet provide clear evidence of lower transfusion exposure in infants. Transfusion outside these algorithms in very preterm infants is not evidence-based and is strongly discouraged.

Best Practices Box

What is the current practice?

Very preterm infants are frequently transfused allogeneic red blood cells according to center-specific clinical practice.

What changes in current practice are likely to improve outcomes?

- A *clinically safe* reduction in transfusion exposure.
- An overarching framework to approach red blood cell transfusion in infants

Is there a Clinical Algorithm?

- Separation of distinct clinical scenarios is essential for transfusion practice in preterm infants.

- For infants with hypovolemic anemia or anemic shock, an approach that considers both clinical and laboratory responses is suggested.

- In contrast, for very low birth weight infants with normovolemic anemia, typically from anemia of prematurity, the use of a restrictive transfusion algorithm based on two recently published trials reduces the transfusion exposure without worsening short or longer term outcomes.

Major Recommendations

- It is recommended that, where possible, clinicians distinguish hypovolemic from normovolemic anemia to inform decisions regarding the timing and volume of transfusion.

- *Prompt restoration of circulating blood volume is critically important in babies with hypovolemic anemia. It is recommended that RBCs are given in aliquots, measuring the effect of each volume on hemodynamic responses (heart rate and blood pressure) and laboratory values (Hb, lactate). This may require transfusion volumes of different sizes delivered over variable time intervals.*

- *Very preterm infants, with normovolemic anemia, usually from anemia of prematurity, should be transfused according to the restrictive arm of either the ETTNO or TOP trials (see* Tables 1–3) *with the volume of transfusion defined by the trial algorithm used.*

Bibliographic Source(s)

- Kirpalani H, Bell EF, Hintz SR, Tan S, Schmidt B, Chaudhary AS, et al. Higher or Lower Hemoglobin Transfusion Thresholds for Preterm Infants. N Engl J Med. 2020;383(27):2639-51.

- Franz AR, Engel C, Bassler D, Rudiger M, Thome UH, Maier RF, et al. Effects of Liberal vs Restrictive Transfusion Thresholds on Survival and Neurocognitive Outcomes in Extremely Low-Birth-Weight Infants: The ETTNO Randomized Clinical Trial. JAMA. 2020;324(6):560-70.

DISCLOSURE

The authors have nothing to disclose.

REFERENCES

1. Keir AK, Yang J, Harrison A, et al. Temporal changes in blood product usage in preterm neonates born at less than 30 weeks' gestation in Canada. Transfusion 2015;55(6):1340–6.
2. Adamson SK Jr, Gandy GM, James LS. The Influence of thermal factors upon oxygen consumption of the newborn human infant. J Pediatr 1965;66:495–508.
3. Sauer PJ, Dane HJ, Visser HK. New standards for neutral thermal environment of healthy very low birthweight infants in week one of life. Arch Dis Child 1984;59(1): 18–22.
4. Chapman CE, Stainsby D, Jones H, et al. Ten years of hemovigilance reports of transfusion-related acute lung injury in the United Kingdom and the impact of preferential use of male donor plasma. Transfusion 2009;49(3):440–52.
5. Stainsby D, Jones H, Asher D, et al. Serious hazards of transfusion: a decade of hemovigilance in the UK. Transfus Med Rev 2006;20(4):273–82.
6. Stramer SL, Dodd RY, Subgroup D. Transfusion-transmitted emerging infectious diseases: 30 years of challenges and progress. Transfusion 2013;53(10 Pt 2): 2375.
7. Duke T. Dysoxia and lactate. Arch Dis Child 1999;81(4):343–50.

8. Van Ameringen MR, Fouron JC, Bard H etal. Oxygenation in anaemic newborn lambs with lambs with high or low affinity red cells. Pediatr Res 1981;15:1500–3.

9. Stockman JA 3rd, Clark DA. Weight gain: a response to transfusion in selected preterm infants. Am J Dis Child 1984;138(9):828–30.

10. Alverson DC, Isken VH, Cohen RS. Effect of booster blood transfusions on oxygen utilization in infants with bronchopulmonary dysplasia. J Pediatr 1988; 113(4):722–6.

11. Poets CF, Pauls U, Bohnhorst B. Effect of blood transfusion on apnoea, bradycardia and hypoxaemia in preterm infants. Eur J Pediatr 1997;156(4):311–6.

12. Wardrop CA, Holland BM, Veale KE, et al. Nonphysiological anaemia of prematurity. Arch Dis Child 1978;53(11):855–60.

13. Mally P, Golombek SG, Mishra R, et al. Association of necrotizing enterocolitis with elective packed red blood cell transfusions in stable, growing, premature neonates. Am J Perinatol 2006;23(8):451–8.

14. Vamvakas EC. White-blood-cell-containing allogeneic blood transfusion and postoperative infection or mortality: an updated meta-analysis. Vox Sang 2007; 92(3):224–32.

15. Mohamed A, Shah PS. Transfusion associated necrotizing enterocolitis: a meta-analysis of observational data. Pediatrics 2012;129(3):529–40.

16. Kirpalani H, Zupancic JA. Do transfusions cause necrotizing enterocolitis? The complementary role of randomized trials and observational studies. Semin Perinatol 2012;36(4):269–76.

17. Cooke RW, Drury JA, Yoxall CW, et al. Blood transfusion and chronic lung disease in preterm infants. Eur J Pediatr 1997;156(1):47–50.

18. Keyes WG, Donohue PK, Spivak JL, et al. Assessing the need for transfusion of premature infants and role of hematocrit, clinical signs, and erythropoietin level. Pediatrics 1989;84(3):412–7.

19. DeMaio JG, Harris MC, Deuber C, et al. Effect of blood transfusion on apnea frequency in growing premature infants. J Pediatr 1989;114(6):1039–41.

20. Bifano EM, Smith F, Borer J. Relationship between determinants of oxygen delivery and respiratory abnormalities in preterm infants with anemia. J Pediatr 1992; 120(2):292–6.

21. Delivoria-Papadopoulos M, Miller LD, Forster RE 2nd, et al. The role of exchange transfusion in the management of low-birth-weight infants with and without severe respiratory distress syndrome. I. Initial observations. J Pediatr 1976;89(2):273–8.

22. Dani C, Reali M, Bertini G, et al. The role of blood transfusions and iron intake on retinopathy of prematurity. Early Hum Dev 2001;62(1):57–63.

23. Silvers K, Gibson A, Russell J, et al. Antioxidant activity, packed cell transfusions, and outcome in premature infants. Arch Dis Child Fetal Neonatal Ed 1998;78(3): F214–9.

24. Hay S, Zupancic JA, Flannery DD, et al. Should we believe in transfusion-associated enterocolitis? Applying a GRADE to the literature. In: Seminars in perinatology41. WB Saunders; 2017. p. 80–91.

25. Rogers SC, FTt Moynihan, McDonough R, et al. Effect of plasma processing and storage on microparticle abundance, nitric oxide scavenging, and vasoactivity. Transfusion 2019;59(S2):1568–77.

26. Thomas KA, Shea SM, Yazer MH, et al. Effect of leukoreduction and pathogen reduction on the hemostatic function of whole blood. Transfusion 2019;59(S2): 1539–48.

27. Wood A, Wilson N, Skacel P, et al. Reducing donor exposure in preterm infants requiring multiple blood transfusions. Arch Dis Child Fetal Neonatal Ed 1995; 72(1):F29–33.

28. da Cunha DH, dos Santos N, Kopelman BI. etal. Transfusions of CPD-1 red blood cells stored for up to 28 days decrease donor exposure in very low-birth-weight premature infants. Transfus Med 2005;15(6):467–73.

29. Foukaneli T, Kerr P, Bolton-Maggs PHB, et al. Guidelines on the use of irradiated blood components. Br J Haematol 2020;191(5):704–24.

30. Kopolovic I, Ostro J, Tsubota H, et al. A systematic review of transfusion-associated graft-versus-host disease. Blood. The Journal of the American Society of Hematology 2015;126(3):406–14.

31. Saito-Benz M, Sandle ME, Jackson PB, et al. Blood transfusion for anaemia of prematurity: current practice in Australia and New Zealand. J Paediatr Child Health 2019;55(4):433–40.

32. Guillén Ú, Cummings JJ, Bell EF, et al. International survey of transfusion practices for extremely premature infants. In: Seminars in perinatology36. WB Saunders; 2012. p. 244–7.

33. McGoldrick E, Stewart F, Parker R, et al. Antenatal corticosteroids for accelerating fetal lung maturation for women at risk of preterm birth. Cochrane Database Syst Rev 2020;12(12):CD004454.

34. Carson JL, Guyatt G, Heddle NM, et al. Clinical practice guidelines from the AABB: red blood cell transfusion thresholds and storage. JAMA 2016;316(19): 2025–35.

35. National Blood Authority C, Australia. Patient Blood Management guidelines: Module 6 - Neonatal and Paediatrics. 2016.

36. Stainsby D, Russell J, Cohen H, et al. Reducing adverse events in blood transfusion. Br J Haematol 2005;131(1):8–12.

37. Cain SM. Oxygen delivery and uptake in dogs during anemic and hypoxic hypoxia. J Appl Physiol Respir Environ Exerc Physiol 1977;42(2):228–34.

38. Andersen C, Karayil S, Hodyl N, et al. Early red cell transfusion favourably alters cerebral oxygen extraction in very preterm newborns. Arch Dis Child Fetal Neonatal Ed 2015;100(5):F433–5.

39. Andersen CC, Keir AK, Kirpalani HM, et al. Anaemia in the premature infant and red blood cell transfusion: new approaches to an age-old problem. Current Treatment Options in Pediatrics 2015;1:191–201.

40. Lumb AB, Thomas CR. Nunn's applied respiratory physiology eBook. Elsevier Health Sciences; 2020.

41. Simmonds MJ, Detterich JA, Connes P. Nitric oxide, vasodilation and the red blood cell. Biorheology 2014;51(2–3):121–34.

42. Schulze A, Whyte RK, Way RC, et al. Effect of the arterial oxygenation level on cardiac output, oxygen extraction, and oxygen consumption in low birth weight infants receiving mechanical ventilation. J Pediatr 1995;126(5 Pt 1):777–84.

43. Krogh A, Lindhard J. The regulation of respiration and circulation during the initial stages of muscular work. J Physiol 1913;47(1–2):112–36.

44. Adams RP, Dieleman LA, Cain SM. A critical value for O2 transport in the rat. J Appl Physiol Respir Environ Exerc Physiol 1982;53(3):660–4.

45. Van Ameringen MR, Fouron JC, Bard H, et al. Oxygenation in anemic newborn lambs with high or low oxygen affinity red cells. Pediatr Res 1981;15(12):1500–3.

46. Yoshida T, AuBuchon J, Tryzelaar L, et al. Extended storage of red blood cells under anaerobic conditions. Vox Sang 2007;92(1):22–31.

47. Fergusson DA, Hebert P, Hogan DL, et al. Effect of fresh red blood cell transfusions on clinical outcomes in premature, very low-birth-weight infants: the ARIPI randomized trial. JAMA 2012;308(14):1443–51.
48. Spinella PC, Tucci M, Fergusson DA, et al. Effect of fresh vs standard-issue red blood cell transfusions on multiple organ dysfunction syndrome in critically ill pediatric patients: a randomized clinical trial. JAMA 2019;322(22):2179–90.
49. Treleaven J, Gennery A, Marsh J, et al. Guidelines on the use of irradiated blood components prepared by the British Committee for Standards in Haematology blood transfusion task force. Br J Haematol 2011;152(1):35–51.
50. Moroff G, Holme S, AuBuchon JP, et al. Viability and in vitro properties of AS-1 red cells after gamma irradiation. Transfusion 1999;39(2):128–34.
51. Saito-Benz M, Bennington K, Gray CL, et al. Effects of freshly irradiated vs irradiated and stored red blood cell transfusion on cerebral oxygenation in preterm infants: a randomized clinical trial. JAMA Pediatr 2022;176(5):e220152.
52. Saito-Benz M, Murphy WG, Tzeng YC, et al. Storage after gamma irradiation affects in vivo oxygen delivery capacity of transfused red blood cells in preterm infants. Transfusion 2018;58(9):2108–12.
53. Meier J, Kemming GI, Kisch-Wedel H, et al. Hyperoxic ventilation reduces six-hour mortality after partial fluid resuscitation from hemorrhagic shock. Shock 2004;22(3):240–7.
54. Cibulskis CC, Maheshwari A, Rao R, et al. Anemia of prematurity: how low is too low? J Perinatol 2021;41(6):1244–57.
55. Widness JA. Pathophysiology of anemia during the neonatal period, including anemia of prematurity. NeoReviews 2008;9(11):e520–5.
56. Kirpalani H, Bell EF, Hintz SR, et al. Higher or lower Hemoglobin transfusion thresholds for preterm infants. N Engl J Med 2020;383(27):2639–51.
57. Kirpalani H, Whyte RK, Andersen C, et al. The Premature Infants in Need of Transfusion (PINT) study: a randomized, controlled trial of a restrictive (low) versus liberal (high) transfusion threshold for extremely low birth weight infants. J Pediatr 2006;149(3):301–7.e3.
58. Franz AR, Engel C, Bassler D, et al. Effects of liberal vs restrictive transfusion thresholds on survival and neurocognitive outcomes in extremely low-birth-weight infants: the ETTNO randomized clinical trial. JAMA 2020;324(6):560–70.
59. Connelly RJ, Stone SH, Whyte RK. Early vs. late red cell transfusion in low birth weight infants 986. Pediatr Res 1998;43(4):170.
60. Chen H-L, Tseng H-I, Lu C-C, et al. Effect of blood transfusions on the outcome of very low body weight preterm infants under two different transfusion criteria. Pediatrics & Neonatology 2009;50(3):110–6.
61. Bell EF, Strauss RG, Widness JA, et al. Randomized trial of liberal versus restrictive guidelines for red blood cell transfusion in preterm infants. Pediatrics 2005;115(6):1685–91.
62. Blank JP, Sheagren TG, Vajaria J, et al. The role of RBC transfusion in the premature infant. Am J Dis Child 1984;138(9):831–3.
63. Collins R, Bowman L, Landray M, et al. The magic of randomization versus the myth of real-world evidence. N Engl J Med 2020;382(7):674–8.
64. IntHout J, Ioannidis JP, Borm GF, et al. Small studies are more heterogeneous than large ones: a meta-meta-analysis. J Clin Epidemiol 2015;68(8):860–9.
65. Andersen CC, Stark MJ, Whyte RK, et al. Low versus high haemoglobin concentration threshold for blood transfusion for preventing morbidity and mortality in very low birth weight infants. Cochrane Database Syst Rev 2011;(11):CD000512.

Prophylactic Platelet Transfusions: Why Less Is More

Hilde van der Staaij, MD[a,b,c,*],
Simon J. Stanworth, MA, FRCP (Paeds, UK), PhD, FRCPath[d],
Susanna F. Fustolo-Gunnink, MD, PhD[a,b,c]

KEYWORDS

- Infant • Newborn • Premature • Platelet transfusion • Thrombocytopenia
- Hemorrhage

KEY POINTS

- Three neonatal platelet transfusion trials show no benefit or to varying degrees evidence of harm when applying more liberal platelet transfusion policies.
- We recommend the use of restrictive platelet transfusion thresholds, although recognizing important limitations of these trials.
- Implementation strategies are required to support evidence-based transfusion practices.
- Future research should address the mechanisms of transfusion-related harm and develop more individualized platelet transfusion guidelines.

INTRODUCTION

On March 4, 1908, a term neonate received a blood transfusion for the first time[1]. Since then, the use of blood transfusion components in neonates has steadily increased and has also been adopted into the care of increasingly preterm infants. Platelet transfusions are the second most commonly transfused blood product in neonates, mostly provided with the aim to prevent bleeding, as prophylaxis. In the past, much of the evidence for the safety and efficacy of administering platelets to neonates has been derived from randomized clinical trials (RCTs) in adult patients, often with hematological malignancies, without formal investigation in neonates. This is important, because

a Department of Pediatrics, Division of Neonatology, Willem-Alexander Children's Hospital, Leiden University Medical Center, Albinusdreef 2, 2333 ZA, the Netherlands; b Sanquin Research & Lab Services, Sanquin Blood Supply Foundation, Amsterdam, Plesmanlaan 125, 1066 CX, the Netherlands; c Department of Pediatric Hematology, Emma Children's Hospital, Amsterdam University Medical Center, Meibergdreef 9, 1105 AZ Amsterdam, the Netherlands; d NHSBT, Oxford University Hospitals, NHS Foundation Trust, Radcliffe Department of Medicine, University of Oxford, Headley Way, Headington, Oxford OX3 9DU, United Kingdom
* Corresponding author. Department of Pediatrics, Division of Neonatology, Leiden University Medical Center, Albinusdreef 2, 2333 ZA Leiden, the Netherlands
E-mail address: h.van_der_staaij@lumc.nl

Clin Perinatol 50 (2023) 775–792
https://doi.org/10.1016/j.clp.2023.07.007
0095-5108/23/© 2023 Elsevier Inc. All rights reserved.

perinatology.theclinics.com

it became increasingly clear that the neonatal hemostatic system differs from that of adults.[2]

When considering the relative benefits and risks of platelets, it should be recognized that all blood components are biological products with risks of transfusion-associated adverse events (eg, transfusion-transmitted infection or transfusion-associated circulatory overload [TACO]) or those related to administration errors. In addition, platelets are recognized to have functions beyond primary hemostasis including inflammatory and immunologic effects, and it has been hypothesized that there is a developmental mismatch between immature neonatal platelets and adult donor platelets, which may have clinical consequences.[3–5]

The first platelet transfusion trial in neonates was published in 1993.[6] This trial aimed to investigate whether early treatment of thrombocytopenia (when platelet counts dropped below 150×10^9/L) would decrease the incidence or extension of intracranial hemorrhage (ICH) compared with initiating treatment at a severe thrombocytopenia threshold of 50×10^9/L. Years after this, in 2019, two other trials have been published comparing restrictive versus liberal transfusion thresholds in preterm neonates.[7,8] These studies recommended the use of lower platelet transfusion thresholds, but the optimal thresholds are still unknown, and there is persistent and widespread variation in clinical practice.

With the publication of the 2-year neurodevelopmental follow-up of the Platelets for Neonatal Transfusion-2/Management of Thrombocytopenia in Special Subgroup (PlaNeT-2/MATISSE) trial and recent publications about variation in neonatal transfusion practice,[9–11] it is time to review the trials and long-term follow-up data, address their limitations, and discuss the challenges and implications for practice and research.

PLATELET TRANSFUSION TRIALS IN PRETERM NEONATES

Three platelet transfusion trials have been conducted to inform the risk–benefit balance for different prophylactic platelet transfusion strategies in preterm neonates. In **Table 1**, we provided an overview of the most relevant trial characteristics and the main results on bleeding, mortality, and neurodevelopmental and respiratory endpoints. We summarized the screening and selection process and the baseline characteristics of these trials in **Fig. 1** and **Table 2**, respectively.

In 1993, Andrew and colleagues performed the first platelet transfusion trial in neonates.[6] The trial compared a liberal (150×10^9/L) versus a restrictive (50×10^9/L) platelet count transfusion threshold to investigate new-onset or extension of ICH (based on the Papile classification[12]). The cohort consisted of 152 preterm neonates with a gestational age (GA) less than 33 weeks and birth weight between 500 and 1500 g. Neonates with initial platelet counts less than 50×10^9/L were excluded. Platelet counts of neonates in the liberal group were maintained greater than 150×10^9/L until day 7 of the study by a maximum of one to three platelet transfusions, whereas infants in the restrictive group did not receive a platelet transfusion unless their platelet count fell to less than 50×10^9/L, or if the infant was bleeding. Cranial ultrasound scans were performed before treatment and repeated on day 7 to 10 of the study. The follow-up was complete for 91% of the neonates. The incidence of new ICH or an existing bleed becoming more extensive was comparable between both groups. However, there was a higher increase in the number of major ICH in the liberal compared with the restrictive group (see **Table 1**). It should be acknowledged that neonatal practice has changed considerably since babies were recruited into this trial, and of course, neonatal intensive care units (NICUs) are now supporting much younger GA infants.

Table 1
Platelet transfusion trials in preterm neonates

	Andrew et al,[6] 1993	Kumar et al,[7] 2019	Curley et al,[8] 2019
Location	4 NICUs in Canada	1 NICU in India	43 NICUs in United Kingdom, Ireland, and the Netherlands
Recruitment period	3-y period (years not specified)	March 2016–April 2017	June 2011–August 2017
Inclusion criteria	• GA <33 weeks • Birth weight 500–1500 g • Platelet count <150 × 10⁹/L in the first 72 h of life with initial platelet count ≥50 × 10⁹/L	• GA <35 weeks • Hemodynamically significant PDA detected at <14 d of postnatal age • Platelet count <100 × 10⁹/L	• GA <34 weeks • Cranial ultrasonography showing no major IVH within 6 h before randomization • Platelet count <50 × 10⁹/L
N total included	152	44	660
Intervention	liberal (150 × 10⁹/L) vs restrictive (50 × 10⁹/L) threshold	liberal (100 × 10⁹/L) vs restrictive (20 × 10⁹/L) threshold[a]	liberal (50 × 10⁹/L) vs restrictive (25 × 10⁹/L) threshold
Primary endpoint	New onset or extension of ICH up to day 10 of life	Time between randomization and closure of PDA during study period of 120 h	Composite of death or major bleeding up to day 28 after randomization
Bleeding endpoints	New or more extensive ICH[b]: 28.2% (liberal) vs 25.7% (restrictive), P = .73 Proportion of infants who developed a grade III or IV ICH[c] 15.4% (liberal) vs 6.8% (restrictive)	Any grade IVH: 40.9% (liberal) vs 9.1% (restrictive), P = .034 Major IVH (grade III/IV): 18.2% (liberal) vs 9.1% (restrictive) P = .6	Major bleeding or mortality[b]: 26% (liberal) vs 19% (restrictive) OR 1.57 (95% CI 1.06–2.32), P = .02 At least one major bleed through trial day 28: 14% (liberal) vs 11% (restrictive) HR 1.32 (95% CI 1.00–1.74)
Mortality endpoints	11 infants (7.2%) died before reaching day 7–10 of the study (not stratified by intervention arm)	Mortality during study period: 31.8% (liberal) vs 36.4% (restrictive), P = .9 Mortality during hospital stay: 36.4% (liberal) vs 40.9% (restrictive), P = .9	Death through trial day 28 15% (liberal) vs 10% (restrictive) OR 1.56 (95% CI 0.95–2.55)

(continued on next page)

Table 1
(continued)

	Andrew et al,[6] 1993	Kumar et al,[7] 2019	Curley et al,[8] 2019
Respiratory endpoints	N/A	N/A	BPD at 36 weeks of PMA: 63% (liberal) vs 54% (restrictive) OR 1.54 (95% CI 1.03–2.30)
Neurodevelopmental outcomes at 2 y of corrected age	N/A	N/A	Death up to 2 y or unfavorable outcome[d]: 50% (liberal) vs 39% (restrictive) OR 1.54 (1.09–2.17), $P = .0167$
Respiratory outcomes at 2 y of corrected age	N/A	N/A	Death or respiratory support required at 2 y: 38% (liberal) vs 28% (restrictive) OR 1.62 (95% CI 1.12–2.34) Respiratory support required at 2 y (excluding deaths): 11% (liberal) vs 4% (restrictive) OR 2.86 (95% CI 1.25–6.51)

Abbreviations: BPD, bronchopulmonary dysplasia; GA, gestational age; HR, hazard ratio; ICH, intracranial hemorrhage; IVH, intraventricular hemorrhage; N/A, not available; OR, odds ratio; PDA, patent ductus arteriosus; PMA, postmenstrual age.

[a] Depending on clinical criteria: $<20 \times 10^9$/L in non-bleeding neonates, $<50 \times 10^9$/L before a major non-neurosurgical intervention, $<100 \times 10^9$/L before a neurosurgical intervention.

[b] Primary outcome.

[c] Calculations based on Table 2 of Andrew et al: 15.4% ([24/78]–[12/78]) and 6.8% ([14/74]–[9/74]).

[d] Unfavorable outcome defined as cerebral palsy that impaired independent walking; global developmental delay assessed by health care professionals as >9 mo behind expected for age; severe seizure disorder; hearing impairment not correct by hearing aids; or bilateral visual impairment with no useful vision (light perception only).

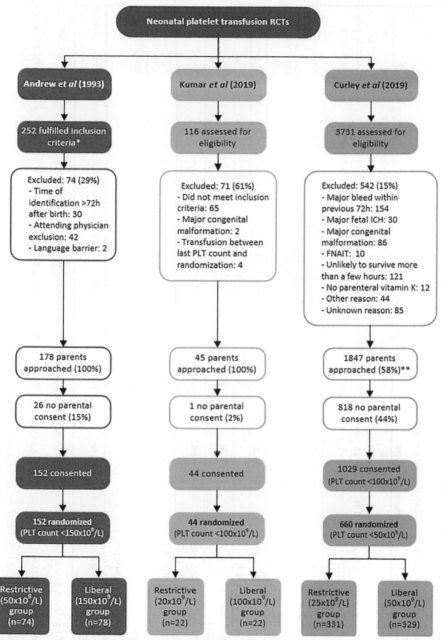

Fig. 1. Screening and selection process of the platelet transfusion trials in neonates. PLT, platelet; ICH, intracranial hemorrhage; FNAIT, fetal and neonatal alloimmune thrombocytopenia. *The total number of neonates checked for eligibility is not reported. **Parents of 1342 neonates were not approached: 559 infants had a PLT count recovery $\geq 100 \times 10^9$/L before consent, 108 parents were too upset to discuss research, 65 stayed too briefly in hospital to permit recruitment, 122 were missed, 348 had another reason, and 140 had an unknown reason.

Table 2
Baseline characteristics of platelet transfusion trials in preterm neonates

	Andrew et al,[6] 1993		Kumar et al,[7] 2019		Curley et al,[8] 2019	
	Restrictive (50 × 10⁹/L) group (n = 74)	Liberal (150 × 10⁹/L) group (n = 78)	Restrictive (20 × 10⁹/L)[a] group (n = 22)	Liberal (100 × 10⁹/L) group (n = 22)	Restrictive (25 × 10⁹/L) group (n = 331)	Liberal (50 × 10⁹/L) group (n = 329)
Gestational age in weeks, mean ± SD or median (IQR)	27.7 ± 2.5	27.4 ± 2.2	30.0 ± 2.0	29.3 ± 2.4	26.7 (24.9–28.7)	26.6 (24.9–28.9)[b]
Birth weight in grams, mean ± SD or median (IQR)	931 ± 266	915 ± 235	1149.1 ± 303.1	1074.7 ± 307.5	743 (605–990)	728 (600–940)[b]
Median weight in grams at randomization (IQR)	N/A	N/A	1060 (913–1275)	984 (808–1171)	892 (670–1190)[c]	860 (668–1170)
Male sex, n(%)	40 (54.0)	49 (62.8)	13 (59.1)	11 (50.0)	191 (57.7)	205 (62.5)[b]
Cesarean delivery, n(%)	N/A	N/A	12 (54.5)	9 (40.9)	201 (61.0)	208 (63.0)[b]
Median postnatal age in days at randomization (IQR)	1.6 (N/A)	1.9 (N/A)	3.0 (2.0–4.2)	3.0 (2.0–4.2)	7.0 (3.7–18.9)	8.4 (4.0–21.0)[b]
Median platelet count (x10⁹/L) at enrollment (IQR)	115 (N/A)	111 (N/A)	68 (47–92)	66 (46–91)	38 (28–44)	38 (29–44)[b]
Treatment for NEC at enrollment, n(%)	1 (1.4)	3 (3.8)	N/A	N/A	49 (14.8)	58 (17.7)[b]
Antibiotic treatment for (suspected) sepsis at enrollment, n(%)	N/A	N/A	2 (9.0)	1 (4.5)	206 (62.2)	209 (63.7)[b]
Existing major IVH at enrollment, n(%)	9 (12.2)	12 (15.4)	N/A	N/A	40 (12.1)	39 (11.9)[b]

Abbreviations: Major IVH defined, as intraventricular hemorrhage (IVH) filling at least 50% of a cerebral ventricle; IQR, interquartile range; Major, IVH; N/A, not available; NEC, necrotizing enterocolitis.
[a] Depending on clinical criteria: <20 × 10⁹/L in non-bleeding neonates, <50 × 10⁹/L before a major non-neurosurgical intervention, <100 × 10⁹/L prior to a neurosurgical intervention.
[b] Data were missing for one infant in the liberal threshold group.
[c] Data were missing for one infant in the restrictive threshold group.

A trial by Kumar and colleagues compared a liberal platelet count threshold of 100×10^9/L to a restrictive threshold in which platelet concentrates were transfused per standard criteria: (1) platelet count less than 20×10^9/L, (2) clinical bleed (ie, any visible fresh oral, nasal, endotracheal, gastrointestinal, or skin bleed), (3) platelet count less than 50×10^9/L before a major non-neurosurgical intervention, or (4) less than 100×10^9/L before a neurosurgical intervention.[7] The primary outcome was time to patent ductus arteriosus (PDA) closure and secondary outcomes included new-onset intraventricular hemorrhage (IVH) of any grade and major (grade III/IV) IVH during the study period. The study population consisted of 44 preterm neonates with a GA less than 35 weeks and a hemodynamically significant PDA detected in the first 2 weeks of life. In the liberal group, two platelet transfusions were administered when the platelet count dropped below 50×10^9/L and one platelet concentrate when the platelet count ranged between 50 and 100×10^9/L. The follow-up time was fixed at 5 days for all study participants. Severe IVH was reported to occur in 18% versus 9% of infants in the liberal versus restrictive group, respectively. The incidence of any IVH grade was significantly higher in the liberal group compared with the restrictive group (see **Table 1**). As for the study by Andrew and colleagues, these differences in outcomes of bleeding should be interpreted with caution given the sample size of the trial.

Finally, the PlaNeT-2/MATISSE trial (2019) compared a liberal (50×10^9/L) versus a restrictive (25×10^9/L) platelet count threshold in 660 infants with a GA less than 34 weeks.[8] The primary outcome was a composite of death or major bleeding up to and including day 28. The follow-up was complete for 99% of the neonates. The study showed increased rates of mortality and major bleeding in the liberal versus the restrictive arm. A secondary analysis indicated that the benefit of a restrictive threshold was evident in all neonates, irrespective of their predicted baseline risk of major bleeding and/or mortality.[13] Furthermore, in the liberal group, a higher incidence of the secondary outcome bronchopulmonary dysplasia (BPD) was observed (see **Table 1**). A post hoc analysis of the composite outcome of death or BPD (to allow for deaths before a possible diagnosis of BPD) yielded a similar odds ratio. There was no difference in the secondary outcomes necrotizing enterocolitis (NEC), sepsis, and retinopathy of prematurity.

Parent and public input into neonatal trials have consistently emphasized the importance of longer term neurodevelopmental follow-up. A further publication from the PlaNeT-2/MATISSE research team reported on 2-year follow-up outcomes. In this study, data were obtained for the majority of PlaNeT-2/MATISSE participants (92%) to assess their neurodevelopmental outcomes at a corrected age of 2 years, using a composite of death or unfavorable outcome (ie, neurodevelopmental impairment [NDI] defined as >9 months behind expected for age, cerebral palsy, seizure disorder, profound hearing or vision loss) as a prespecified outcome.[9] Three clinicians, who were blinded for the treatment arm, independently evaluated all available information and reported the outcome on a standardized 2-year outcome form. Using a mixed logistic regression model, the study found that the higher platelet transfusion threshold of 50×10^9/L increased the rate of death or severe NDI at a corrected age of 2 years. However, as only 41% of the children received a formal neurodevelopmental assessment, subtle outcome differences could not be detected. In addition, given the initial finding of a higher incidence of BPD in the liberal threshold group, a post hoc analysis was performed to evaluate the proportion of participants who had died or were dependent on oxygen or respiratory support at 2 years of corrected age, showing a higher need for respiratory support at 2 years among children randomized to the 50×10^9/L threshold group (see **Table 1**).

CHALLENGES IN PLATELET TRANSFUSION TRIALS

The use of randomized controlled trials has been a cornerstone in the development and evaluation of new or existing therapies for preterm infants. However, despite the fact that the platelet trials were designed to minimize bias and test different treatment decisions, they can come with challenges and limitations, which should be considered in the context of implementation of results. In **Table 3**, we discuss several epidemiologic challenges in neonatal transfusion RCTs and consider some of these points from the perspective of the platelet transfusion trials.

One of the main challenges is variation in treatment intervention (including standard of care) between trials, and sometimes also within trials, for instance in multicenter settings. Treatment variation in platelet transfusion trials can occur at several levels. For example, there can be differences in administration (eg, dose and rate) and donor/donation characteristics, such as product specifications (eg, irradiation, pathogen inactivation technologies, storage duration, and differences in the degree of ABO blood group (in)compatibility). As a result of this variation, different trials, and sometimes even different centers within the same trial, are in fact testing different treatments. In general, data on donor and product characteristics are often not readily available to neonatologists. To facilitate assessment of trial generalizability, the intervention under evaluation should be clearly defined and consistent as far as possible within and across trials, including data on component specifications, transfusion volume, and duration.

A further challenge is variation in outcome definitions, including use of composite outcomes, nonformal assessment of long-term outcomes, and definitions of adverse events. Composite outcomes are commonly used in neonatal trials, but there is extensive literature describing the pros and cons of such outcomes.[14,15] Guidelines for the use of composite outcomes suggest that each component should be equally severe and aligned in the same direction of effect, because if the components of the primary outcome change in opposite directions then no effect might be observed, despite a clinically important difference between treatments. An example of this related to platelet transfusion trials is the use of the composite death or an unfavorable outcome at 2 years of corrected age in the PlaNeT-2/MATISSE follow-up, in which NDI may not be considered equally severe as death.[9] In addition, the study was not powered for the long-term follow-up outcome and several assessment tools were used to assess NDI, which also included non-validated tools such as whether the treating physician deemed a child to be impaired, which hampered evaluation of more subtle neurodevelopmental outcome differences. This pragmatic approach to use whatever data are available is understandable, often given the financial and logistical challenges of conducting long-term follow-up studies, but should be recognized, and discussed when developing these studies. Last, in neonatal transfusion trials, adverse effects are often not well-defined and mostly reported at the discretion of neonatologists. We need to improve more neonatal specific definitions for transfusion-associated adverse events, such as transfusion-related acute lung injury, transfusion-related acute lung injury (TACO), and transfusion-associated dyspnea (TAD), and report these in future trials.

Third, pre-randomization transfusions, protocol violations, and lack of blinding are study conduct-related issues that often occur. Pre-randomization transfusions are common in neonatal transfusion trials as a result of a delay caused by the informed consent procedure or babies not being identified on time as eligible for the trial, and possibly also some unease in the mind of attending neonatologists about potential delays to platelet transfusion, particularly in very preterm neonates just after birth. In the PlaNeT-2/MATISSE trial, 39% of the infants received a platelet transfusion before

Table 3
Epidemiologic challenges in neonatal transfusion randomized clinical trials

Issues in/between trial(s)	Examples	Potential Solutions for Future Studies
Between trial and within trial variation in interventions	Differences in: • Donor characteristics • Transfusion product specifications • Transfusion dose and rate • Threshold definitions	• Describe the intervention in a clear and consistent way, including data on component specifications, transfusion volume, and duration
Between trial and within trial variations in outcome definitions	• Incorrect use of composite outcomes • Non-formal assessment of long-term outcomes • Lack of definitions for transfusion-associated adverse events	• Use standardized and objective outcome measures • Reconsider the use of composite outcomes or improve their composition • Perform separate power calculations for long-term outcomes • Improve definitions for neonatal transfusion-associated adverse events and report these in future trials
Study conduct issues	• Pre-randomization transfusions • Protocol violations • Lack of blinding • Inappropriate exclusions	• Facilitate randomization at an early postnatal age by improving consenting procedures • Perform a sensitivity analysis in case of considerable pre-randomization transfusions • Improve protocol adherence in future trials • Record other treatments that might be adjusted based on the assigned transfusion thresholds to evaluate the presence of post-randomization bias
Generalizability/external validity	• Important patient (sub)groups not included in the trials • Relatively high number of parental consent refusals for their child's participation in RCTs	• Choose a study population that is representative of the target population, including analyses to assess heterogeneity of treatment effect • Collaborate with parent representatives of preterm or ill-born neonates • Repeat trials in other settings, including important subgroups (eg, surgical/ECMO patients) that have not yet been evaluated in other trials

Abbreviations: RCTs, randomized controlled trials; ECMO, extracorporeal membrane oxygenation.

randomization (121 in the restrictive group and 126 in the liberal group).[8] These pre-randomization transfusions might affect the trial generalizability and may dilute the treatment effect, as it is possible that these transfusions were given during the highest risk period for ICH. Some of these infants may never have developed platelet counts less than 50×10^9/L after the initial transfusion and were therefore excluded from the trial. Facilitating randomization at an early postnatal age by improving consenting and screening procedures should therefore be a priority in future trials. Additional analyses of the trial data could be performed to investigate the extent to which those transfusions might have impacted the observed treatment effect.

Protocol violations with disbalance between the arms increase the risk of bias toward the null and platelet count separation between trial arms does not guarantee sufficient contrast between the study arms, as in all trials platelet count measurements were done at the discretion of the treating neonatologist. These implications for the PlaNeT-2/MATISSE trial might be limited, as a difference between the arms was still observed despite protocol violations.[8]

The lack of blinding may allow clinicians to adjust the management of neonates consciously or unconsciously depending on the trial arm in which the neonate was randomized, potentially leading to post-randomization bias. However, blinded studies in transfusion are practically very difficult to execute. Future studies should focus on the development of standardized and objective outcome measures and record other treatments that might be adjusted based on the assigned transfusion thresholds to evaluate the presence of post-randomization bias.

Finally, the external validity of neonatal platelet transfusion trials is limited to neonates with comparable characteristics to the study populations. In the PlaNeT-2/MATISSE trial, neonates with early-onset thrombocytopenia (ie, in the first 72 hour after birth) were recruited but perhaps underrepresented. Further important patient (sub)groups that have not been assessed in the trials are neonates with a GA at birth $\geq$35 weeks, neonates with major congenital malformations, those who undergo invasive procedures or surgery, extracorporeal membrane oxygenation (ECMO) patients, neonates with a family history of or confirmed fetal neonatal alloimmunre thrombocytopenia (FNAIT), and actively bleeding neonates. Furthermore, there were a total of 381 neonates in the trials whose parents/guardians were not approached for study participation because they were missed or for unknown reasons, and of the 2070 parents/guardians who were approached, 41% did not provide consent (see **Fig. 1**). Efforts to improve screening for eligibility and optimization of consent procedures are necessary to exclude infants for no other reasons than the prespecified exclusion criteria and to obtain consent as early as possible. Collaboration with parent representatives of preterm or ill-born neonates could help identify barriers for study participation, which could then be addressed to minimize selection bias due to consent refusal.

In summary, future studies might consider these trial design points to help develop more robust studies, alongside general recommendations for the reporting of randomized trials. Other areas to consider, beyond the scope of this review, include analysis plans. Additional subgroup analyses could be performed to assess heterogeneity of treatment effect, such as has been performed for the PlaNeT-2/MATISSE study.[13]

WHAT IS THE EVIDENCE ON UPTAKE OF RESEARCH FINDINGS INTO NEONATAL PRACTICE?

To evaluate the extent to which the results of the platelet transfusion trials reflect and/or have changed platelet transfusion practices in neonatal care, we now summarize the results of two recently published studies about neonatal platelet transfusion practices in the United States and Europe, respectively.

Patel and colleagues described in a retrospective cohort study the incidence of blood product transfusions in neonates, including platelet transfusions, using data from seven North American tertiary and quaternary NICUs between 2013 and 2016.[10] All birth admissions during the study period of the participating sites were included, resulting in a total cohort of 60.243 infants. Ninety percent of this cohort consisted of term infants ($\geq$37 weeks' gestation), with 329 neonates with a GA less than 27 weeks. The incidence of platelet transfusions was 0.7% (95% CI 0.6%–0.7%) among the full cohort and 35% (95% CI 29%–39%) among preterm infants less than 27 weeks' gestation. The median pre-transfusion platelet count was 71×10^9/L (10th–90th percentile $26-135 \times 10^9$/L) for the entire cohort, 85×10^9/L (17–185) for term infants, and 70×10^9/L (33–100) for infants with a GA less than 27 weeks, though this included presurgery thresholds. The highest median pre-transfusion platelet counts ($>100 \times 10^9$/L) were observed among neonates receiving ECMO for congenital diaphragmatic hernia and/or persisting pulmonary hypertension of the newborn. No distinction could be made between prophylactic transfusions and those administered in response to clinically significant bleeding. This study demonstrated wide variability in neonatal platelet transfusion practices in the United States, with a large proportion of transfusions administered at thresholds higher than currently supported by the best available evidence. Importantly, the study assessed clinical data from before the publication of the PlaNeT-2/MATISSE trial. Several subsequent implementation studies in NICUs in the United States and Canada have been published,[16–18] suggesting that the clinical thresholds may have been lowered since then, though epidemiologic data are lacking.

Scrivens and colleagues also reported substantial ongoing variation in platelet transfusion practices across European centers based on an online survey performed among 597 NICUs in 18 European countries with care for infants less than 32 weeks' gestation.[11] This study was coordinated by the Neonatal Transfusion Network, a recently established international, interdisciplinary research network dedicated to neonatal transfusion research (see https://neonataltransfusionnetwork.com/). The survey included NICUs in the period from October to December 2020, which was 2 years after the publication of the PlaNeT-2/MATISSE trial. In this Survey on Transfusion practices among European Preterm infants admitted to Neonatal Intensive Care Units (STEP), 47% to 57% of the NICUs indicated using platelet transfusion thresholds above 25×10^9/L in non-bleeding neonates. For infants who received ibuprofen for PDA treatment, thresholds $\geq25 \times 10^9$/L were used in 84% of the NICUs. Thresholds $\leq20 \times 10^9$/L were used in 27% and 34% of the NICUs for infants with a GA less than 28 weeks and 28 to 32 weeks without bleeding, respectively. In addition to thresholds, there was widespread variation in transfusion volume and duration. National guidelines have been changed to adopt the restrictive platelet count thresholds of 25×10^9/L in at least the United Kingdom and the Netherlands,[19] but this survey showed that on a European scale transfusion thresholds still tend to be more liberal compared with the recommended restrictive threshold based on the PlaNeT-2/MATISSE results,[8] highlighting that this is an important area for further research. A prospective, international, multicenter observational point prevalence study is ongoing and includes data from more than 75 NICUs from 22 European countries, to gain more insight into current neonatal transfusion practices.[20]

In **Fig. 2**, we created a boxplot based on the data of both studies to show the variation in platelet count transfusion thresholds stratified by GA in the US-based and European NICUs. As the two studies presented their data in different ways, we could not

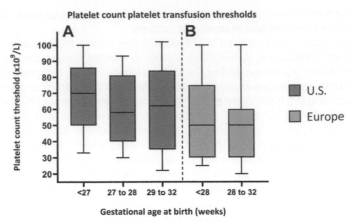

Fig. 2. Boxplot showing the variation in platelet count transfusion thresholds by gestational age in (*A*) US-based NICUs and (*B*) European NICUs. The boxplot's extreme whiskers represent the 10th and 90th percentiles. (*Data from* Patel and colleagues *J. Pediatr.* 2021 and Scrivens and colleagues *Arch Dis Child Fetal Neonatal Ed.* 2023.[10,11])

take into account the variation in transfusion thresholds for different clinical scenarios of thrombocytopenia (eg, surgery, lumbar puncture, ibuprofen) and for transfusions given either prophylactically or in response to bleeding. Although the figure might appear to suggest that higher thresholds are used in the United States compared with Europe, the US data were collected before the publication of the PlaNeT-2/MATISSE trial. The main message of the figure is that it highlights considerable variation in platelet transfusion practice and the need to better understand implementation of neonatal platelet transfusion research findings into clinical practice.[21]

DISCUSSION

In this review, we have summarized the three neonatal platelet transfusion trials, which included a total of 856 neonates. The studies showed no benefit with more liberal platelet transfusion thresholds, and—all to varying degrees—demonstrated some evidence of harm including an increased risk of major bleeding or death associated with the use of more liberal platelet transfusion thresholds. On the other hand, we have identified and discussed potentially important shortcomings and challenges for neonatal platelet transfusion trials.

Recommendations

Despite the limitations of the trials, given the severity of the reported transfusion-related harm and the lack of evidence of benefit for the liberal transfusion thresholds—including 2-year neurodevelopmental outcomes—our overall view is that the trials support the use of restrictive platelet transfusion thresholds. **Box 1** provides a summary of our suggested restrictive policies for platelet transfusions based on the thresholds as tested in the randomized trials. **Box 2** provides a response to common concerns with regard to the recent trials and implementation into clinical practice. Future full systematic reviews, additional analyses and follow-up studies of existing trials, new randomized trials, and complementary observational and translational studies are required to come to more robust recommendations.

In addition, we recommend informing parents about the complexity and uncertainties of transfusion decisions and involving them in the decision-making process.

Box 1	
Recommended platelet transfusion thresholds	
Patient group	**Platelet count threshold**
• Non-bleeding preterm neonates (gestational age <37 weeks) not scheduled to undergo an invasive procedure	• 25 × 10^9/L
• Neonates scheduled to undergo an invasive procedure, who are actively bleeding, or who have experienced major bleeding within the last 72 h	• No recommendation, as these groups were included in trials, but additional transfusions were allowed at the discretion of the treating neonatologist. Current consensus-based guidelines suggest thresholds varying between 50 and 100 × 10^9/L
• Neonates with a major congenital malformation	• No recommendation, as these neonates were excluded from all trials

Of note:
• Any threshold *above the highest recommended* is not evidence-based.
• Any threshold *below the lowest recommended* has not yet been tested (clinical equipoise).

The risk of drafting clinical guidelines with scarce evidence is that this uncertainty is not conveyed to health care professionals, and as a result, is not fully explained to parents. Parents have a right to be made aware of clinical uncertainty and should be informed about the potential benefits and risks of transfusions. In case of clinical equipoise or lack of evidence, their opinion on whether or not their child should receive a blood transfusion becomes even more pivotal.

Future Research Directions

Perhaps one of the bigger challenges in neonatal transfusion medicine is that the platelet transfusion trials were designed as parallel arm studies, comparing only two threshold interventions. Therefore, clinicians are still left without an answer as to what is the optimal threshold for prophylactic platelet transfusions (eg, possibly a threshold of 10 × 10^9/L or lower). Future clinical transfusion trials might benefit from more innovative designs, such as data-driven embedded trials, adaptive trials, and platform trials. Such studies could also explore the safety of much lower thresholds, for example, platelet counts less than 10 × 10^9/L which are less commonly seen in practice. In addition to clinical trials, we need a strong emphasis on observational studies and large vein-to-vein data sets to explore associations between donor and product characteristics and clinical outcomes and to benchmark and monitor current practice.

Furthermore, two neonates with similar platelet counts but different clinical conditions may have distinct risks of bleeding and may benefit differently from platelet transfusions. Platelet count-based transfusion thresholds do not accurately identify neonates whose bleeding or death could be prevented by a platelet transfusion from those in which a prophylactic transfusion likely has no effect or might even lead to transfusion-associated adverse events. Incorporating a more personalized approach, for example, by using risk-based thresholds with the use of a validated dynamic prediction model for major bleeding that includes multiple clinical variables in addition to platelet count may perform better and thereby improve patient outcomes.[22] Alternatively, a whole blood test of primary hemostasis, such as the Platelet Function Analyzer Closure Time in response to Collagen and adenosine diphosphate

---

Box 2
Common concerns regarding platelet transfusion trials and implementation into clinical practice

- **Concern 1: Are the results of the trials valid?**
  We have reviewed the three neonatal platelet transfusion trials and conclude that there are several common limitations among all trials. However, we do consider these trials to be the best evidence currently available to guide clinical transfusion decisions. Future new trials and systematic reviews can be consulted to hopefully verify our findings.

- **Concern 2: I am not certain the results of the trial are generalizable to my center/country.**
  The effects of transfusions will depend on different patient, donor, NICU, product, and administration characteristics. Some of these variables can be compared between the trial population and individual centers or countries, such as neonatal baseline characteristics. Some of the product characteristics are also made explicit in trial publications and could be verified for centers/countries. Unfortunately, for most other variables, it is unknown how and to what extent these differ between the trial populations and individual centers or countries. This makes it difficult to assess whether the trial results may or may not apply, and underlines the need for more studies describing these variables in both the study populations and general neonatal populations. In the meantime, you will have to navigate this uncertainty by estimating to what extent these variables may differ between your center and the trial populations, and to what extent this may affect the outcome of the transfusion strategy. In the absence of the evidence needed to make this assessment, unless there are very strong arguments against this, following the trial recommendations may be the most appropriate strategy.

- **Concern 3: I am not certain the results of the trial apply to a particular subgroup of neonates.**
  Whether the trial results apply to specific subgroups is always a difficult question to answer, because by definition we do not know the answer, as trials are not usually powered for subgroup analyses. As an example, in the PlaNeT-2/MATISSE trial, one of the issues raised in recent opinion papers was the relative lack of early-onset thrombocytopenia in the trial population, as 37% of neonates were randomized before day 5 of life. Some institutions and individual researchers have therefore made an exception in the implementation of the trial results, allowing for higher transfusion thresholds in the first few days of life. This concern is understandable and underlines the need for further studies; however, in our opinion, the translation of subgroup concerns into clinical practice guidelines requires careful assessment of several questions. We have considered these questions for the specific example of early-onset thrombocytopenia in the PlaNeT-2/MATISSE trial.
  1. To what extent is the subgroup represented in the trial? The subgroup is underrepresented: 37% were randomized before the 5th day of life, this should have been around 55% based on Dutch and UK observational studies (Fustolo-Gunnink et al Haematologica. 2019, Figure S3, and Stanworth et al Pediatrics. 2009): median postnatal age of 4 days at first platelet count $<60 \times 10^9$/L, that is, at least 50% of severe thrombocytopenia within the first 4 days of life.[22,23]
  2. Are there signals in the trial that hint at a different effect in the subgroup? No, both the conventional subgroup analysis in the primary paper and a more advanced analysis published separately do not suggest a differential transfusion effect in the first few days of life.[13]
  3. Are there signals in other studies or plausible biological pathways that would justify different treatment in the subgroup? No, to our knowledge, there are no studies that show a differential effect of transfusions depending on postnatal age. The hemostatic system will be more immature in the early days of life, potentially exaggerating the developmental mismatch, but the implications of this mismatch are unknown.[5] The incidence of major bleeding is higher in the first days of life, but this does not imply that transfusions will be (more) effective in preventing these bleeds.
  4. What are the risks of transfusing versus not transfusing in this subgroup?
     - Risk of not transfusing: it is possible that platelet transfusions sometimes, in some neonates, prevent major bleeding. The problem is that we cannot identify these children with our current evidence base.

- Risk of transfusing: 7% overall absolute increase in risk of major bleeding and/or mortality. Within the subgroup of neonates with postnatal age <72 hours at randomization, the risk difference is 14%, though this analysis is underpowered, as mentioned previously.
  Our view is that in the specific case of early-onset thrombocytopenia in the PlaNeT-2/MATISSE trial, the weight of the trial results outweighs the risks of a potential differential effect of treatment in this subgroup. We encourage clinicians to address concerns about other subgroups in a similarly structured way.

- **Concern 4: What should be the lowest thresholds for platelet transfusions?**
  The STEP survey indicated that 27% to 34% of the NICUs use platelet thresholds lower than those tested in PlaNeT-2/MATISSE. These NICUs are now faced with the question of whether they should increase their transfusion thresholds. We argue that from a purely scientific point of view, because the lower thresholds have not yet been tested, there is clinical equipoise and therefore clinicians can choose whether or not to transfuse more restrictively. The question is not whether severe thrombocytopenia is harmful to a preterm infant, the question is whether platelet transfusions can mitigate this harm, and whether transfusion-related adverse events outweighs any beneficial effects. As a historical example, in the PlaNeT-1 study, an observational study describing platelet transfusion practices in the United Kingdom, 42% of transfusions were administered at a minimum platelet count of $<25 \times 10^9$/L, which was lower than the recommended thresholds at the time.[23] If this had not been the case, recruitment for the PlaNeT-2/MATISSE trial might have been extremely difficult. In this case, variation in clinical practice was beneficial to the design and conduct of new trials. On the other hand, from an educational/implementation perspective, it may be preferable to define a temporary lower transfusion threshold while awaiting new randomized trials. We suggest that this threshold should be based not only on the trials but also on current clinical practice and could therefore be lower than the lowest ranges tested in the trials.

(ADP), is a promising approach to better predict which babies are more likely to bleed, although the relatively high blood volumes (800 μL) required for this currently hamper its widespread use in the neonatal population.[23] New platelet parameters (eg, immature platelet fraction) are being investigated as markers of bleeding risk in thrombocytopenic preterm neonates, which can be measured simultaneously with platelet count without the need for additional blood.[24] It is essential to conduct quantitative and qualitative studies to investigate differences in clinical context that may explain or justify the use of different transfusion strategies and to understand the barriers and facilitators to translating research findings into clinical practice. Consequently, targeted, tailored implementation studies could help reduce the current evidence-to-practice gap and may be used for the development of improved and individualized guidelines on platelet transfusion in neonates.

Last, the reasons for the observed higher incidence of major bleeding or mortality in the liberal arm of the PlaNeT-2/MATISSE trial are still unknown. Several potential mechanisms of harm have been proposed. First, preterm infants generally receive much higher transfusion volumes compared with adults, circa 15 mL/kg compared with 5 mL/kg, respectively.[11] The rapid volume expansion after administration of a platelet transfusion may induce hemodynamic shifts that could contribute to an increased risk of hemorrhage by disturbing the blood flow in the brain at the location of the germinal matrix. Second, there likely is a developmental mismatch, as there are considerable differences between adult and premature neonatal platelets, including adult platelets being functionally hyperreactive compared with neonatal platelets, but we do not yet fully understand the implications of this mismatch.[5,25,26] Finally, our understanding of the functions of platelets has improved considerably over the last few decades and has revealed a complex interplay between the cellular and noncellular components of the blood and the immunologic and inflammatory pathways.[2,4] Therefore, it is plausible that transfusion-associated adverse events are (at least in part) related to the immunologic and/or inflammatory properties of platelets.

Because it is very difficult to predict what will happen to adult platelets once they are introduced into a premature neonatal circulatory system, we need high-quality basic research studies to better understand the pathophysiology of neonatal thrombocytopenia and the effects of platelet transfusions. More fundamental and translational research is essential to elucidate the underlying mechanisms of transfusion-related harm to help physicians more accurately determine the risks/benefits of platelet transfusions in thrombocytopenic preterm neonates.

SUMMARY

In short, given the current evidence base, we recommend the use of restrictive platelet transfusion thresholds while awaiting the results of new/ongoing studies and large-scale epidemiologic studies. Future trialists will have an opportunity to address the identified challenges and additionally improve the efficiency and design of these trials using electronic patient data and advanced trial designs. There clearly is a need for new biomarkers and models to better predict bleeding risk for more tailored platelet transfusion decisions, implementation strategies to support evidence-based transfusion practices, and fundamental research to better understand the mechanisms of transfusion-related harm.

Best Practices Box

What is the current practice for neonatal thrombocytopenia?

There is a widespread variation in platelet transfusion practices for the management of neonatal thrombocytopenia. Three platelet transfusion trials in preterm neonates showed no benefit with higher transfusion thresholds. The most recent trial (PlaNeT-2/MATISSE) demonstrated an increased risk of major bleeding or mortality when applying more liberal transfusion policies, with a higher rate of death or significant neurodevelopment impairment at a corrected age of 2 years.

What changes in current practice are likely to improve outcomes?

Despite the potentially important shortcomings of the neonatal platelet transfusion trials and the challenges of translating these research findings into neonatal practice, we believe that they support the paradigm shift from "*better safe than sorry*" to "'*less is more.*'" While awaiting the results of new/ongoing studies to address the identified challenges in neonatal transfusion trials (**Table 3** and **Box 2**) and to better understand the mechanisms of transfusion-related harm, following the recommendations of the PlaNeT-2/MATISSE trial is likely the most appropriate strategy to improve neonatal outcomes.

Major recommendations

- Given the severity of the reported transfusion-associated harm and the lack of evidence of benefit for the liberal transfusion thresholds, we recommend the use of restrictive platelet transfusion thresholds in neonates (see **Box 1**).

Bibliographic sources

- Andrew M, Vegh P, Caco C, et al. A randomized, controlled trial of platelet transfusions in thrombocytopenic premature infants. J Pediatr. 1993;123(2):285 to 291.

- Curley A, Stanworth SJ, Willoughby K, et al. Randomized Trial of Platelet-Transfusion Thresholds in Neonates. N Engl J Med. 2019;380(3):242 to 251.
- Kumar J, Dutta S, Sundaram V, Saini SS, Sharma RR, Varma N. Platelet Transfusion for PDA Closure in Preterm Infants: A Randomized Controlled Trial. Pediatrics. 2019;143(5).

DISCLOSURE

S.J. Stanworth and S.F. Fustolo-Gunnink were involved in the PlaNeT-2/MATISSE trial and STEP survey. H. van der Staaij has nothing to disclose.

REFERENCES

1. Raju TNK. Historical perspectives: cured by the blood: the story of the first neonatal blood transfusion. NeoReviews 2006;7(2):e67–8.
2. Ferrer-Marín F, Sola-Visner M. Neonatal platelet physiology and implications for transfusion. Platelets 2022;33(1):14–22.
3. Stolla M, Refaai MA, Heal JM, et al. Platelet transfusion - the new immunology of an old therapy. Front Immunol 2015;6:28.
4. McFadyen JD, Kaplan ZS. Platelets are not just for clots. Transfus Med Rev 2015; 29(2):110–9.
5. Davenport P, Sola-Visner M. Hemostatic challenges in neonates. Front Pediatr 2021;9:627715.
6. Andrew M, Vegh P, Caco C, et al. A randomized, controlled trial of platelet transfusions in thrombocytopenic premature infants. J Pediatr 1993;123(2):285–91.
7. Kumar J, Dutta S, Sundaram V, et al. Platelet transfusion for PDA closure in preterm infants: a randomized controlled trial. Pediatrics 2019;143(5).
8. Curley A, Stanworth SJ, Willoughby K, et al. Randomized trial of platelet-transfusion thresholds in neonates. N Engl J Med 2019;380(3):242–51.
9. Moore CM, D'Amore A, Fustolo-Gunnink S, et al. Two-year outcomes following a randomised platelet transfusion trial in preterm infants. Arch Dis Child Fetal Neonatal Ed 2023.
10. Patel RM, Hendrickson JE, Nellis ME, et al. Variation in neonatal transfusion practice. J Pediatr 2021;235:92–9.e94.
11. Scrivens A, Reibel NJ, Heeger L, et al. Survey of transfusion practices in preterm infants in Europe. Archives of Disease in Childhood - Fetal and Neonatal Edition. 2023:fetalneonatal-2022-324619.
12. Papile LA, Burstein J, Burstein R, et al. Incidence and evolution of subependymal and intraventricular hemorrhage: a study of infants with birth weights less than 1,500 gm. J Pediatr 1978;92(4):529–34.
13. Fustolo-Gunnink SF, Fijnvandraat K, van Klaveren D, et al. Preterm neonates benefit from low prophylactic platelet transfusion threshold despite varying risk of bleeding or death. Blood 2019;134(26):2354–60.
14. Montori VM, Permanyer-Miralda G, Ferreira-González I, et al. Validity of composite end points in clinical trials. BMJ 2005;330(7491):594–6.
15. Cordoba G, Schwartz L, Woloshin S, et al. Definition, reporting, and interpretation of composite outcomes in clinical trials: systematic review. BMJ 2010;341:c3920.
16. Davenport PE, Chan Yuen J, Briere J, et al. Implementation of a neonatal platelet transfusion guideline to reduce non-indicated transfusions using a quality improvement framework. J Perinatol 2021;41(6):1487–94.

17. Bahr TM, Christensen TR, Henry E, et al. Platelet transfusions in a multi-neonatal intensive care unit health care organization before and after publication of the PlaNeT-2 clinical trial. J Pediatr 2023;257:113388.
18. Zabeida A, Chartrand L, Lacroix J, et al. Platelet transfusion practice pattern before and after implementation of a local restrictive transfusion protocol in a neonatal intensive care unit. Transfusion 2023;63(1):134–42.
19. New HV, Stanworth SJ, Gottstein R, et al. British Society for Haematology Guidelines on transfusion for fetuses, neonates and older children. Br J Haematol 2020; 191(5):725–7 (Br J Haematol. 2016;175:784-828). Addendum August 2020.
20. Houben NAM, et al. Observational study of blood transfusions in European preterm infants (INSPIRE study). Updated: December 2, 2022; In: ISRCTN Registry: ISRCTN17267090, Available at: https://www.isrctn.com/ISRCTN17267090. Accessed: May 30, 2023.
21. Sola-Visner M, Leeman KT, Stanworth SJ. Neonatal platelet transfusions: new evidence and the challenges of translating evidence-based recommendations into clinical practice. J Thromb Haemost 2022;20(3):556–64.
22. Fustolo-Gunnink SF, Fijnvandraat K, Putter H, et al. Dynamic prediction of bleeding risk in thrombocytopenic preterm neonates. Haematologica 2019;104(11):2300–6.
23. Deschmann E, Saxonhouse MA, Feldman HA, et al. Association of bleeding scores and platelet transfusions with platelet counts and closure times in response to adenosine diphosphate (CT-ADPs) among preterm neonates with thrombocytopenia. JAMA Netw Open 2020;3(4):e203394.
24. Deschmann E, et al. The Neonatal Hemorrhagic Risk Assessment in Thrombocytopenia (NEOHAT-2). Updated: March 22, 2023; In: ClinicalTrials.gov identifier: NCT04598750, Available at: https://clinicaltrials.gov/ct2/show/NCT04598750. Accessed: May 30, 2023.
25. Ferrer-Marin F, Chavda C, Lampa M, et al. Effects of in vitro adult platelet transfusions on neonatal hemostasis. J Thromb Haemost 2011;9(5):1020–8.
26. Liu ZJ, Italiano J Jr, Ferrer-Marin F, et al. Developmental differences in megakaryocytopoiesis are associated with up-regulated TPO signaling through mTOR and elevated GATA-1 levels in neonatal megakaryocytes. Blood 2011;117(15): 4106–17.

Hemostatic and Immunologic Effects of Platelet Transfusions in Neonates

Patricia Davenport, MD[a],*, Erin Soule-Albridge, MS[b],
Martha Sola-Visner, MD[c]

KEYWORDS

- Neonate • Platelets • Platelet transfusion • Immunology • Hemostasis

KEY POINTS

- Liberal platelet transfusions are associated with increased morbidity and mortality among preterm neonates admitted to the neonatal intensive care unit.
- Platelets are known to have both hemostatic and immune functions.
- Neonatal platelets are hypo-reactive to multiple platelet agonists compared with adult platelets, but little is known regarding differences in platelet immune function across development.
- The harm associated with neonatal platelet transfusions might be due to alterations in the neonatal hemostatic balance or abnormal immune responses induced by the presence of adult platelets.

INTRODUCTION

As discussed elsewhere in this issue, 3 randomized platelet transfusion threshold trials in preterm neonates have been published to date, with all three finding no evidence of benefit from liberal transfusions in decreasing the incidence of bleeding.[1–3] Furthermore, two of the 3 trials found an increase in morbidity and/or mortality among neonates randomized to the higher platelet count thresholds, compared with the lower threshold.[2,3] More recently, a long-term follow-up study of children previously included in the PlaNeT-2 trial reported a higher incidence of death or poor neurodevelopmental outcomes at 2 years of age among children randomized to the liberal compared with the restrictive platelet transfusion threshold, raising the possibility that platelet transfusions might also affect the developing brain.[4]

[a] Division of Newborn Medicine, Boston Children's Hospital, 300 Longwood Avenue, Enders 954, Boston, MA 02115, USA; [b] Division of Newborn Medicine, Boston Children's Hospital, 300 Longwood Avenue, Enders 950.5, Boston, MA 02115, USA; [c] Division of Newborn Medicine, Boston Children's Hospital, 300 Longwood Avenue, Enders 961, Boston, MA 02115, USA
* Corresponding author.
E-mail address: Patricia.Davenport@childrens.harvard.edu

Clin Perinatol 50 (2023) 793–803
https://doi.org/10.1016/j.clp.2023.07.002
0095-5108/23/© 2023 Elsevier Inc. All rights reserved.
perinatology.theclinics.com

The mechanisms mediating these deleterious effects are unknown, but it has been hypothesized that they could be related to the increasingly recognized nonhemostatic functions of platelets and to the developmental differences that exist between adult (transfused) and neonatal platelets. This article reviews the current understanding of these differences and the hemostatic and immunologic effects of platelet transfusions in neonates.

RESEARCH
Nonhemostatic Functions of Platelets

Platelets are the primary hemostatic cells in circulation and are critical to control bleeding. Historically, this was thought to be the only function of platelets, but it is now clear that platelets are key participants in multiple nonhemostatic processes, including the inflammatory response, response to infection, vascular growth, vascular tone, and tumor biology (**Fig. 1**).[5-7] A study investigating the mRNA profile of neonatal and adult platelets found that the biologic processes most enriched in platelets from both neonates and adults were involved in immune functions, further supporting this paradigm shift in platelet biology.[8] It has now been demonstrated that platelets interact with the immune system in multiple ways and play anti-infective, proinflammatory, and immunoregulatory roles (**Table 1**).

To help defend the host from infection, platelets express pattern recognition receptors including toll-like receptors (TLR4, TLR2, TLR6, and TLR7),[9] C-type lectin receptors (CLEC-2 and DC-Sign),[10] and NOD-like receptors (NLRs),[11] through which they recognize damage-associated molecular patterns (DAMPs) and pathogen-associated molecular patterns (PAMPs).[12] Signaling through these receptors triggers the production and release of inflammatory cytokines and antimicrobial molecules

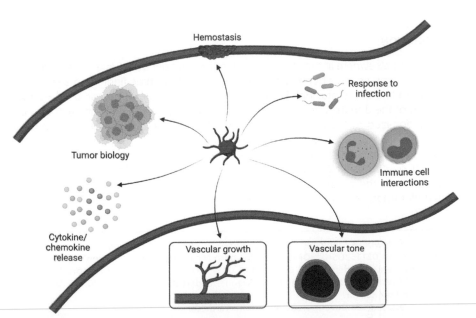

Fig. 1. Platelets have multiple functions beyond their roles in hemostasis, including antimicrobial functions, interactions with immune cells, cytokine/chemokine release, and regulation of vascular tone, vascular growth, and tumor biology.

Table 1
Platelet immune functions and cellular interactions

Category	Type of Platelet Immune Interaction/Function	Details
Anti-infective	Platelet pattern recognition receptors	Toll-like Receptors (TLR4, TLR2, TLR1, TLR6, and TLR7)
		C-type lectin receptors (CLEC-2 and -DC-Sign)
		NOD-like receptors (NOD2 and NLRP3)
	Platelet-derived antimicrobial molecules	β-defensins
		α-defensins
		Thrombocidins
		IL-1β
Immunoregulatory	Release of platelet-derived soluble immune mediators	CD40L
		PF4 (CXCL4)
		RANTES (CCL5)
		NAP-2 (CXCL-7)
		B-2 microglobulin (β-2M)
	Platelet leukocyte aggregate formation	Platelet neutrophil aggregate formation
		Platelet monocyte aggregate formation
	Platelet regulation of monocyte functions	Regulation of monocyte inflammatory phenotype
		Regulation of monocyte migratory phenotype
	Platelets and complement	Platelets contain C3, C4a, C1-inhibitor, and factor H
	Platelets and APCs	Multiple interactions with dendritic cells
	Platelets and T-cells	Recruit T-cells to vascular injury and promote differentiation
	Platelets as APCs	Platelets express approximately 80,000 MHC-I molecules on the surface
	Platelet Fc receptor	Platelets express FcγRIIa receptor
	Platelets and NK cells	Platelets recruit NK cells to vascular injury
	Platelets and B-cells	Multiple B-cell interactions involving the CD40L/CD40 axis
	Platelet-derived microvesicles	The most abundant microvesicles in circulation

Abbreviations: APCs, antigen presenting cells; MHC, major histocompatibility complex; NK, natural killer.

from platelets, the interaction of platelets with immune cells, and the binding of platelets to invading organisms.

Platelets can interact with immune cells, including neutrophils and monocytes through either cell-cell interactions or through the release of soluble mediators stored in the platelet granules or translated in response to specific signals. Upon activation, platelets express multiple ligands on their surface, including P-selectin, and release soluble immune mediators including soluble CD40 ligand (sCD40L), platelet factor 4 (PF4 or CXCL4), RANTES (CCL5), NAP-2 (CXCL7), and β-2 microglobulin (β-2M).[5] Once P-selectin is expressed on the surface, it is available to bind to its receptor, PSGL-1, found on the surface of immune cells including neutrophils and monocytes.[13,14] These platelet-leukocyte aggregates are then able to enhance platelet activation, increase neutrophil and monocyte activation/mobilization, and increase monocyte Mac-1 expression (an integrin crucial for leukocyte recruitment to the endothelium).[13–16]

Different studies have shown that platelets use both of these mechanisms (direct cell-cell interaction and release of mediators) to regulate the monocyte inflammatory response. Thrombin-activated platelets induce the expression and secretion of cytokines (specifically MCP-1 and interleukin [IL]-8) from human monocytes. This response was initially shown to depend on both platelet P-selectin surface exposure and the platelet release of RANTES, as blocking either reversed the findings.[17] More recently, activated platelets were also shown to release β-2M, a molecular chaperone for the major histocompatibility class I (MHC I) complex, which promotes monocyte differentiation towards a pro-inflammatory phenotype. Conversely, TGF-β promotes monocyte differentiation towards a pro-reparative phenotype. Both β2M and TGF-β compete for binding to the TGFBR-1, but signal through different downstream pathways to promote opposite monocyte differentiation paths.[18,19]

In addition to monocytes, platelets interact readily with neutrophils and are able to enhance the release of neutrophil extracellular traps (NETs).[20] NETs are networks of histone-studded DNA released from neutrophils that can bind pathogens in the blood stream.[21] Although NETs are able to trap, fix, and kill pathogens, they also can have deleterious systemic effects by causing vascular occlusion and subsequent organ damage.[22,23] Interestingly, the placenta releases a NET-inhibitory factor to prevent NET formation in utero that can still be detected in the days after birth, thus inhibiting the neonate's ability to make NETs during the first few days of life.[24,25]

In addition to interacting with and contributing to the innate immune system, platelets also interact with and initiate complement activation and are active participants in the adaptive immune system.[12] Platelets can initiate the alternative and classic complement pathways through P-selectin activation of C3[26] and binding of C1q,[27] respectively, and assembly of the terminal complement complex (C5b-9) on the platelet surface induces platelet activation and secretion.[28,29] Platelets can also act as antigen-presenting cells, as they have over 80,000 MHC-1 molecules on their surface,[30] and interact with T-cells,[31] B-cells,[32] and NK cells[33] to recruit cells to areas of injury and promote or alter cellular differentiation (see **Table 1**) in a complex and highly context-specific manner. In summary, it is now clear that platelets are both hemostatic and immune cells. However, little is known regarding developmental differences in platelet immune functions and whether/how these differences contribute to the harmful effects of liberal platelet transfusions in neonates.

Developmental differences between neonatal and adult platelets

Multiple studies over the last 3 decades have demonstrated that neonatal platelets are hyporeactive compared with adult platelets in response to most agonists. Following activation with epinephrine, adenosine diphosphate (ADP), thrombin, thromboxane, or collagen (all traditional agonists), neonatal platelets bind less fibrinogen, express less surface P-selectin (a marker of alpha granule degranulation), and exhibit less aggregation than adult platelets activated with the same agonists.[34] Various mechanisms contribute to the hypo-responsiveness of neonatal platelets, including decreased surface expression of some receptors (ie, for epinephrine, thrombin, and collagen), decreased intracellular signaling (for collagen), decreased calcium mobilization (for thromboxane), enhanced sensitivity to inhibitory pathways (PGE-1), and impaired degranulation.[34]

Although the degree of hypo-reactivity of neonatal platelets would predict a clinical bleeding phenotype, studies of whole-blood primary hemostasis, including in vivo bleeding times and in vitro platelet function analyzer (PFA-100) closure times, paradoxically found shorter bleeding and closure times in full-term neonates compared with healthy adults, indicating enhanced neonatal primary hemostasis.[35,36] Preterm neonates have longer bleeding and closure times than term neonates, but they are still well within the normal adult range. The explanation for this paradoxical finding is that the hypo-reactivity of neonatal platelets is well balanced by neonatal factors that promote and accelerate clotting, such as their high hematocrit, high mean corpuscular volume, and high vWF concentrations with a predominance of ultralong polymers.[35,37] Thus, it is now clear that the hypo-reactivity of neonatal platelets does not represent a deficiency or immaturity, but is rather an integral part of a developmentally different but well-balanced neonatal hemostatic system.

Although the developmental differences in platelet hemostatic functions have been extensively studied and are well recognized, understanding of developmental differences regarding the nonhemostatic functions of platelets has lagged behind. In fact, little is known about the angiogenic or immune functions of neonatal compared with adult platelets, although emerging evidence suggests that adult platelets might be more immune-active than neonatal platelets. As already described, activated neonatal platelets express less P-selectin on the surface compared with their adult counterparts, and translocation of P-selectin to the platelet surface is essential to make it available for binding to its receptor, PSGL-1, on immune cells including neutrophils and monocytes. Thus, the presence of higher P-selectin levels on the surface of adult compared with neonatal platelets would predict an enhanced ability of adult platelets to interact with and activate immune cells, potentially triggering or augmenting systemic or localized tissue inflammation (**Fig. 2**).

A few recent studies have compared the mRNA and protein content of neonatal and adult platelets. The first study to address this question found 201 differentially expressed genes, with up-regulation of mRNAs related to protein synthesis, trafficking and degradation in neonatal platelets, and down-regulation of mRNAs related to calcium transport, metabolism, actin cytoskeleton reorganization, and cell signaling.[8] A more recent study also comparing neonatal and adult platelet mRNA profiles identified DEFA3 (encoding human defensing neutrophil peptide 3) and HBG1 (encoding hemoglobin subunit gamma 1) as biomarkers of neonatal megakaryopoiesis, which could potentially differentiate neonatal from adult platelets.[38]

One study compared the proteome of neonatal and adult platelets and found 170 differentially abundant proteins. In this study, neonatal platelets were enriched for proteins involved in mitochondrial energy metabolism, long chain fatty acid metabolism, and iron binding, while adult platelets were enriched in proteins related to the inflammatory response, platelet activation, blood coagulation, and complement activation.[39]

In addition to these human platelet studies, a recent murine study compared mRNA expression between neonatal (P7) and adult platelets and found adult platelets to be

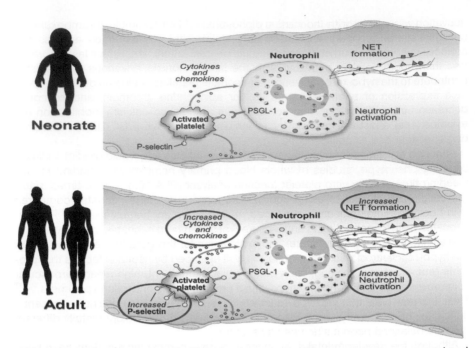

Fig. 2. Schematic representation of key developmental differences between neonatal and adult platelets, and potential effects on immune cells. On activation, human neonatal platelets express less P-selectin and release their alpha granule content (including cytokines and chemokines) less effectively than adult platelets. Decreased P-selectin surface expression results in a reduced ability to interact with and activate immune cells, including neutrophils and monocytes. A neutrophil is shown as an example. The reduced NET formation in neonates is caused by the presence of a placenta-derived NET inhibitor. NET, neutrophil extracellular trap; PSGL-1, P-selectin glycoprotein ligand-1. (*From* Davenport P, Sola-Visner M. Platelets in the neonate: not just a small adult. Res Pract Thromb Haemost 2022;6(3):e12719.)

enriched in mRNAs involved in ubiquitin/proteasome and immune-related pathways.[40] These differences in mRNA and protein content found in people and mice overall support the hypothesis that platelets have different functional specifications at different developmental stages, and that adult platelets might be more immunoactive compared with neonatal platelets.

Effects of Platelet Transfusions on Neonatal Hemostasis and Inflammation

In the context of neonatal platelet transfusions, a key question has been whether transfused adult platelets, which are comparatively hyper-reactive and potentially more immunoactive than neonatal platelets, differentially impact the neonatal hemostatic and immune responses. The first study to address this question generated thrombocytopenic full-term cord blood samples in the laboratory and mixed them with either adult or neonatal platelet concentrates, in order to model in vitro neonatal transfusions with adult or neonatal platelets.[41] As hypothesized, this study showed that transfusion with adult platelets resulted in a significant shortening of the PFA-100 closure times in response to collagen and epinephrine (CT-Epi, an in vitro equivalent to the bleeding time) compared to transfusion with neonatal platelets, to levels that have been associated with an increased risk of cardiovascular events. These findings provided proof of principle for the existence of a potential developmental mismatch associated with the transfusion of adult platelets into the different hemo-static system of neonates, and raised the possibility that platelet transfusions could promote microvascular thrombosis in sick neonates, potentially worsening diseases characterized by tissue ischemia, like necrotizing enterocolitis. However, this remains to be demonstrated in vivo.

Clinically, the hemostatic effectiveness of platelet transfusions, particularly for mod-erate degrees of thrombocytopenia, is rather controversial. One study systematically examined the effects of platelet transfusions on platelet counts, PFA-100 closure times in response to collagen and ADP (CT-ADP), and bleeding scores (to assess the severity of bleeding) in a cohort of 76 neonates with a gestational age less than 32 weeks.[42] This study found that platelet transfusions significantly increased the platelet count and had a small effect shortening the CT-ADP, but did not influence the bleeding score of preterm neonates, suggesting that factors other than the platelet count and/or hemostatic disorders contributed to the bleeding. Consistently, two of the 3 randomized controlled trials published to date reported an increased incidence of bleeding (including IVH) in neonates randomized to the higher platelet transfusion threshold, compared with those transfused at a lower platelet count.[2,3] The reasons underlying this finding are unknown, but it has been hypothesized that they could be related to hemodynamic factors in the setting of transfusing a high volume over a short period of time. Neonates enrolled in PlaNeT-2 received 15 cc/kg of platelets, reflecting standard neonatal practice, usually given over 30 to 60 minutes. This volume is approximately 3 times higher than the 5 cc/kg usually transfused to older children or adults, and it is conceivable that the rapid infusion of such volumes could cause he-modynamic changes leading to bleeding from the fragile germinal matrix vasculature.

Alternatively, recent findings in preclinical models have raised the interesting possi-bility that inappropriate angiogenic signals (ie, originating from transfused hyperactive platelets) during vulnerable developmental periods could lead to dysregulated angio-genesis, formation of aneurysms in the brain, and secondary hemorrhages occurring at mid-gestation, although this remains speculative.[43]

With the growing recognition that platelets are immune cells and that neonatal and adult platelets are developmentally distinct, the inflammatory effects of neonatal platelet transfusions have recently become the subject of research. To determine the inflammatory effect of platelet transfusion in neonates without underlying inflam-mation, the authors' group transfused washed murine adult platelets into postnatal day 10 (P10) pups and found elevated levels of plasma inflammatory cytokines (including IL-6, G-CSF, MCP-1, CXCL-1, IL-1α, IL-1β, and IL-17) 2 and 4 hours after platelet transfusion, compared with buffer transfused controls, suggesting that platelet transfusions can induce an inflammatory response in neonates.[44] To investi-gate the effects of platelet transfusions into a clinically relevant neonatal sepsis model, adult murine platelets were transfused into P10 pups infected with cecal slurry (CS), a model of polymicrobial sepsis. Unexpectedly, platelet transfusions had dual effects on mortality in this model. They increased mortality in septic pups with low baseline mor-tality, but decreased mortality in septic pups with a high baseline mortality.[45] The dele-terious effects of platelet transfusion were accompanied by a global increase in plasma (mostly pro-inflammatory) cytokines, while the beneficial effects of transfusion were associated with a reduction in plasma cytokines. These findings suggested that platelet transfusions can up- or down-regulate neonatal systemic inflammation in response to specific signals, which remain to be identified. Finally, a recent study investigated whether the developmental stage of the transfused platelets (adult versus neonatal) differentially affected the monocyte phenotype of transfused thrombocyto-penic pups (P14). Using in vitro and in vivo models, Maurya and colleagues found that exposure of monocytes to either neonatal or adult platelets increased the percentage of Ly6C[hi] pro-inflammatory monocytes, but only exposure to adult platelets increased the percentage of monocytes displaying a migratory phenotype, characterized by increased surface expression of CCR2 and CCR5 (the receptors for CCL2 and CCL5, respectively). Functionally, the monocytes exposed to adult, but not neonatal, platelets were able to migrate in response to a CCL2 gradient both in vitro and in vivo.[40] Importantly, these findings were partially reversed when P-selectin mediated platelet-monocyte interactions were blocked using a PSGL-1 blocking antibody. Taken together, these findings supported the hypothesis that transfusion of developmentally different platelets (ie, with increased P-selectin surface exposure) could disrupt the neonatal immune balance and lead to dysregulated immune responses, potentially increasing monocyte migration into inflamed tissues.

More research into the immune effects of neonatal platelet transfusions is needed, particularly to unravel the complex effects of platelets in neonates of varying gestational and postnatal ages and with different underlying pathologies, as well as the role of donor, product, and recipient factors on these responses. Nevertheless, the most recent evidence from animal models supports the hypothesis that, similar to the neonatal hemostatic system, neonatal platelets are an integral part of a developmentally unique neonatal immune system (designed to meet the needs of the fetus and neonate), which may be altered by the transfusion of adult platelets that are potentially more pro-inflammatory (**Fig. 3**).

DISCUSSION/FUTURE DIRECTIONS

Platelets have extensive immune functions in addition to their well-described role in hemostasis and are cells that live at the intersection between hemostasis and immunity. Similar to the hemostatic differences between neonatal and adult platelets,

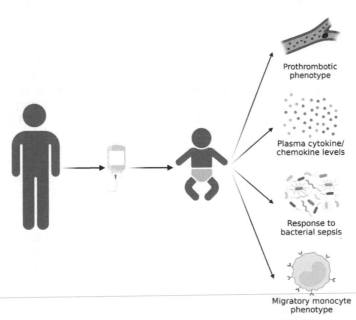

Prothrombotic
phenotype

Plasma cytokine/
chemokine levels

Response to
bacterial sepsis

Migratory monocyte
phenotype

Fig. 3. Hemostatic and immunologic responses affected by platelet transfusions in neonates, based on available in vitro human and in vivo murine studies.

emerging evidence supports that significant developmental differences also exist in regard to the platelet immune functions. In murine models of neonatal thrombocytopenia, the presence of adult platelets, which are potentially more immunoactive than neonatal platelets, can induce dysregulated monocyte migratory responses and induce or modulate systemic inflammation in a highly context-dependent manner. The findings from the PlaNet-2 Trial have made it clear that a change in clinical practice toward the use of evidence-based restricted transfusion protocols and a better understanding of the mechanisms mediating the harm associated with platelet transfusion are needed. Ultimately, this could lead to the development of strategies to block or attenuate the harmful effects of platelet transfusions, while maintaining their hemostatic benefits.

CLINICS CARE POINTS

- Platelets have multiple immune functions.
- Providers should consider the potential for immune/inflammatory effects when ordering a platelet transfusion for a neonate.

DISCLOSURE

The authors have nothing to disclose.

FUNDING

PD: Supported by Program Project Grant (P01) HL046925 (M. Sola-Visner) and K99 HL156051.

REFERENCES

1. Andrew M, Vegh P, Caco C, et al. A randomized, controlled trial of platelet transfusions in thrombocytopenic premature infants. J Pediatr 1993;123:285–91.
2. Kumar J, Dutta S, Sundaram V, et al. Platelet transfusion for PDA closure in preterm infants: a randomized controlled trial. Pediatrics 2019;143:e20182565.
3. Curley A, Stanworth SJ, Willoughby K, et al. Randomized trial of platelet-transfusion thresholds in neonates. N Engl J Med 2019;380:242–51.
4. Moore CM, D'Amore A, Fustolo-Gunnink S, et al. Two-year outcomes following a randomised platelet transfusion trial in preterm infants. Arch Dis Child Fetal Neonatal Ed 2023. https://doi.org/10.1136/archdischild-2022-324915.
5. Maouia A, Rebetz J, Kapur R, et al. The immune nature of platelets revisited. Transfus Med Rev 2020;34:209–20.
6. Koupenova M, Livada AC, Morrell CN. Platelet and megakaryocyte roles in innate and adaptive immunity. Circ Res 2022;130:288–308.
7. Weyrich AS. Platelets: more than a sack of glue. Hematology Am Soc Hematol Educ Program 2014;2014:400–3.
8. Caparros-Perez E, Teruel-Montoya R, Lopez-Andreo MJ, et al. Comprehensive comparison of neonate and adult human platelet transcriptomes. PLoS One 2017;12:e0183042.
9. Cognasse F, Nguyen KA, Damien P, et al. The inflammatory role of platelets via their TLRs and siglec receptors. Front Immunol 2015;6:83.

10. Suzuki-Inoue K, Fuller GL, Garcia A, et al. A novel Syk-dependent mechanism of platelet activation by the C-type lectin receptor CLEC-2. Blood 2006;107:542–9.
11. Zhang S, Zhang S, Hu L, et al. Nucleotide-binding oligomerization domain 2 receptor is expressed in platelets and enhances platelet activation and thrombosis. Circulation 2015;131:1160–70.
12. Elzey BD, Tian J, Jensen RJ, et al. Platelet-mediated modulation of adaptive immunity. A communication link between innate and adaptive immune compartments. Immunity 2003;19:9–19.
13. Kornerup KN, Salmon GP, Pitchford SC, et al. Circulating platelet-neutrophil complexes are important for subsequent neutrophil activation and migration. J Appl Physiol 2010;109:758–67.
14. Freedman JE, Loscalzo J. Platelet-monocyte aggregates: bridging thrombosis and inflammation. Circulation 2002;105:2130–2.
15. Lisman T. Platelet-neutrophil interactions as drivers of inflammatory and thrombotic disease. Cell Tissue Res 2018;371:567–76.
16. Lam FW, Vijayan KV, Rumbaut RE. Platelets and their interactions with other immune cells. Compr Physiol 2015;5:1265–80.
17. Weyrich AS, Elstad MR, McEver RP, et al. Activated platelets signal chemokine synthesis by human monocytes. J Clin Invest 1996;97:1525–34.
18. Hilt ZT, Pariser DN, Ture SK, et al. Platelet-derived beta2M regulates monocyte inflammatory responses. JCI Insight 2019;4:e122943.
19. Hilt ZT, Maurya P, Tesoro L, et al. beta2M signals monocytes through non-canonical TGFbeta receptor signal transduction. Circ Res 2021;128:655–69.
20. Clark SR, Ma AC, Tavener SA, et al. Platelet TLR4 activates neutrophil extracellular traps to ensnare bacteria in septic blood. Nat Med 2007;13:463–9.
21. Vorobjeva NV, Chernyak BV. NETosis: molecular mechanisms, role in physiology and pathology. Biochemistry (Mosc) 2020;85:1178–90.
22. Leppkes M, Knopf J, Naschberger E, et al. Vascular occlusion by neutrophil extracellular traps in COVID-19. EBioMedicine 2020;58:102925.
23. Burmeister A, Vidal YSS, Liu X, et al. Impact of neutrophil extracellular traps on fluid properties, blood flow and complement activation. Front Immunol 2022;13: 1078891.
24. Yost CC, Schwertz H, Cody MJ, et al. Neonatal NET-inhibitory factor and related peptides inhibit neutrophil extracellular trap formation. J Clin Invest 2016;126(10): 3783–98.
25. Yost CC, Cody MJ, Harris ES, et al. Impaired neutrophil extracellular trap (NET) formation: a novel innate immune deficiency of human neonates. Blood 2009; 113:6419–27.
26. Del Conde I, Cruz MA, Zhang H, et al. Platelet activation leads to activation and propagation of the complement system. J Exp Med 2005;201:871–9.
27. Peerschke EI, Yin W, Grigg SE, et al. Blood platelets activate the classical pathway of human complement. J Thromb Haemostasis 2006;4:2035–42.
28. Wiedmer T, Esmon CT, Sims PJ. Complement proteins C5b-9 stimulate procoagulant activity through platelet prothrombinase. Blood 1986;68:875–80.
29. Peerschke EI, Yin W, Ghebrehiwet B. Complement activation on platelets: implications for vascular inflammation and thrombosis. Mol Immunol 2010;47:2170–5.
30. Kao KJ, Cook DJ, Scornik JC. Quantitative analysis of platelet surface HLA by W6/32 anti-HLA monoclonal antibody. Blood 1986;68:627–32.
31. Ponomarev ED. Fresh evidence for platelets as neuronal and innate immune cells: their role in the activation, differentiation, and deactivation of Th1, Th17, and Tregs during tissue inflammation. Front Immunol 2018;9:406.

32. Cognasse F, Hamzeh-Cognasse H, Lafarge S, et al. Human platelets can activate peripheral blood B cells and increase production of immunoglobulins. Exp Hematol 2007;35:1376–87.
33. Maurer S, Ferrari de Andrade L. NK cell interaction with platelets and myeloid cells in the tumor milieu. Front Immunol 2020;11:608849.
34. Ferrer-Marín F, Sola-Visner M. Neonatal platelet physiology and implications for transfusion. Platelets 2022;33(1):14–22.
35. Roschitz B, Sudi K, Kostenberger M, et al. Shorter PFA-100 closure times in neonates than in adults: role of red cells, white cells, platelets and von Willebrand factor. Acta Paediatr 2001;90:664–70.
36. Saxonhouse MA, Garner R, Mammel L, et al. Closure times measured by the platelet function analyzer PFA-100 are longer in neonatal blood compared to cord blood samples. Neonatology 2010;97:242–9.
37. Davenport P, Sola-Visner M. Hemostatic challenges in neonates. Front Pediatr 2021;9:627715.
38. Liu Z, Avila C, Malone LE, et al. Age-restricted functional and developmental differences of neonatal platelets. J Thromb Haemostasis 2022;20:2632–45.
39. Stokhuijzen E, Koornneef JM, Nota B, et al. Differences between platelets derived from neonatal cord blood and adult peripheral blood assessed by mass spectrometry. J Proteome Res 2017;16:3567–75.
40. Maurya P, Ture SK, Li C, et al. Transfusion of adult, but not neonatal, platelets promotes monocyte trafficking in neonatal mice. Arterioscler Thromb Vasc Biol 2023; 43:873–85.
41. Ferrer-Marin F, Chavda C, Lampa M, et al. Effects of in vitro adult platelet transfusions on neonatal hemostasis. J Thromb Haemostasis 2011;9:1020–8.
42. Deschmann E, Saxonhouse MA, Feldman HA, et al. Association of bleeding scores and platelet transfusions with platelet counts and closure times in response to adenosine diphosphate (CT-ADPs) among preterm neonates with thrombocytopenia. JAMA Netw Open 2020;3:e203394.
43. Hoover CKY, Shao B, McDaniel MJ, et al. Heightened activation of embryonic megakaryocytes causes aneurysms in the developing brain of mice lacking podoplanin. Blood 2021;137(20):2756–69.
44. Davenport P, Nolton E, Feldman H, et al. Pro-inflammatory effects of platelet transfusions in newborn mice with and, In: without underlying inflammation. Presented at American Society of Hematology Annual Meeting, held virtually due to COVID-19, 2020.
45. Davenport P, Fan HH, Nolton E, et al. Platelet transfusions in a murine model of neonatal polymicrobial sepsis: divergent effects on inflammation and mortality. Transfusion 2022;62:1177–87.

Blood Donor Sex and Outcomes in Transfused Infants

Anand Salem, DO, Ravi Mangal Patel, MD, MSc*

KEYWORDS

- Red blood cell • Gender • Preterm infant • Blood banking • Transfusion
- Neonatology

KEY POINTS

- Multiple factors related to donor sex may influence the characteristics and quality of transfused red blood cells.
- There are conflicting data from observational studies on the association between the sex of blood donors and outcomes in preterm infants.
- Additional research is needed to elucidate the effect of blood donor characteristics on outcomes in transfused neonates.

INTRODUCTION

Red blood cell (RBC) transfusion is common in the neonatal intensive care, particularly among preterm infants with anemia of prematurity. The incidence of RBC transfusion is 64% among extremely low birth weight (ELBW) infants and 41% among very low birth weight (VLBW) infants.[1] The rationale for RBC transfusion is to treat or prevent potential impairment in oxygen delivery to tissues from anemia by increasing blood oxygen carrying capacity through an increase in hemoglobin. However, RBC transfusions may have effects beyond simply increasing hemoglobin in transfused infants. Prior studies show RBC transfusions in neonates and infants may be pro-inflammatory and cause endothelial activation,[2–4] are major determinants of changes in tissue oxygenation,[5–7] and potentially influence the risk of neonatal diseases, such as bronchopulmonary dysplasia (BPD),[8–10] intestinal injury and necrotizing enterocolitis (NEC),[11–13] and retinopathy of prematurity (ROP).[14,15]

To date, clinical trials have largely focused on comparing the effects of high versus low thresholds for RBC transfusion on clinical outcomes in ELBW or very preterm

Funding: National Institutes of Health K23 HL128942 (R.M. Patel) and Warshaw Fellow Research Award supported by the Emory Department of Pediatrics and Children's Healthcare of Atlanta (A. Salem).
Department of Pediatrics, Emory University and Children's Healthcare of Atlanta, 2015 Uppergate Drive Northeast, Atlanta, GA 30322, USA
* Corresponding author.
E-mail address: rmpatel@emory.edu

Clin Perinatol 50 (2023) 805–820
https://doi.org/10.1016/j.clp.2023.08.001
0095-5108/23/© 2023 Elsevier Inc. All rights reserved.

infants.[16–19] However, these trials have considered all RBC transfusions as a similar exposure. Although most of the trials in neonatal transfusion have studied *when* to transfuse RBCs,[20] there has been less focus on the potential effects of *what* is being transfused (eg, *what* is the bag of the blood unit). Many factors may influence the quality of the RBCs being transfused, including donor characteristics (eg, sex, age), manufacturing characteristics, anticoagulant preservatives, storage, irradiation, volume reduction, aliquoting, and washing (**Fig. 1**).[21] Some of these factors are addressed in another related review article in this issue focused on blood banking practices. In this review article, the authors focus on the potential influence of blood donor sex and related donor characteristics on outcomes among transfused neonates and infants. To identify specific studies and articles relevant to this focus and review, the authors performed a systematic search as detailed below.

SEARCH STRATEGY

To systematically identify studies evaluating the potential impact of blood donor sex on neonates and infants, the authors used the following search strategy without restriction in PubMed (neonat*[tw] OR neo-nat*[tw] OR newborn*[tw] OR new-born*[tw] OR perinat*[tw] OR prematur*[tw] OR Infan*[tw] OR "Infant"[Mesh] OR baby[tw] OR babies[tw]) AND blood[tw] AND donor[tw] AND sex[tw]. The initial search was performed on April 6, 23 and was updated on April 7, 23. The authors identified a total of 185 unique articles, with 178 articles remaining after filtering for English language only. After reviewing the titles, 14 articles were selected for additional abstract review. After reviewing the abstracts of these 14 articles, 8 were excluded. One was excluded because of a focus on plasma transfusion,[22] three were excluded because of a focus on adult patients,[23–25] one for a focus on genetic testing,[26] one for a focus on intrauterine transfusion,[27] and two for a focus on exchange transfusion.[28,29] Among the six articles identified in the search strategy, five reported original findings[30–34] and one was a review article.[35] Details about the five original science articles are summarized in **Table 1** and discussed below.

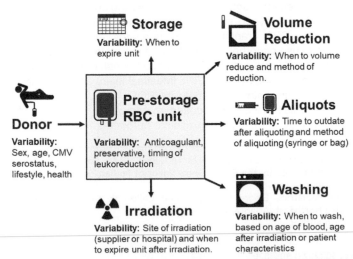

Fig. 1. Potential factors influencing the quality of transfused red blood cells. (*Adapted from* Patel et al.[21])

Table 1
Summary of studies on donor sex and neonatal outcomes

First Author[ref] (Year of Publication)	Type of Study	Population (Sample Size)	Unit of Analysis (Infant or RBC Transfusion Episode)	Primary Comparison	Primary Outcome	Summary of Main Findings
DeSimone et al,[30] 2023	Observational cohort study (secondary analysis)	VLBW infants (≤1500 g) receiving ≥1 RBC transfusion (n = 254 infants, n = 567 un ts)	RBC transfusion episode	RBC units from male donor vs female donor	Posttransfusion hemoglobin increment	Reduced posttransfusion hemoglobin increments were associated with RBC units donated by female donors (−0.24 g/dL; 95% CI −0.57, −0.02; P = .04). For RBC units donated by male donors, reduced donor hemoglobin levels (<13.5 g/dL) were associated with an increased need for subsequent recipient RBC transfusion (odds ratio 3.0; 95% CI 1.3, 6.7; P < .01).

(continued on next page)

Table 1
(continued)

First Author[ref] (Year of Publication)	Type of Study	Population (Sample Size)	Unit of Analysis (Infant or RBC Transfusion Episode)	Primary Comparison	Primary Outcome	Summary of Main Findings
Bahr et al,[31] 2023	Observational cohort study (retrospective)	All neonates receiving ≥1 RBC transfusion (n = 2086 infants, n = 6396 transfusions)	Infant	Infants transfused RBCs from exclusively male donors, exclusively female donors, or from both male and female donors.	Mortality or morbidity (BPD, NEC, ROP)	Infants who received blood from both male and female donors had more RBC transfusions (mean ± SD: 5.3 ± 2.9 transfusions if received both male and female donor blood vs 2.6 ± 2.2 if received blood from only one sex, $P < .001$). There were no significant associations between the sex of the blood donor and the primary outcome (adjusted relative risk of only male vs only female donor 1.05; 95% CI 0.92–1.20; $P = .47$)
Crawford et al,[32] 2023	Observational cohort study (secondary analysis)	Preterm newborns <29 wk gestation (n = 153 infants, n = 367 transfusions)	RBC transfusion episode	Infants receiving RBCs from any female donors, compared with exclusively male	Posttransfusion increases in pro-inflammatory cytokines	Transfusion from female donors was associated with posttransfusion

			increases in pro-inflammatory cytokines (IL-12, IL-17A, IL-6, IL-8, TNF). This relationship seemed related to repeat transfusion exposure (greater with 3rd transfusion). Responses seemed reduced with washed RBCs.
		donors (with washing another factor)	
Patel et al,[33] 2021	Observational cohort study (secondary analysis)	VLBW infants (≤1500 g) receiving ≥1 RBC transfusion (n = 181 infants, n = 499 transfusions)	Infant	Infants transfused RBCs from exclusively from male donors or exclusively from female donors	Mortality or morbidity (BPD, NEC, ROP)	In multivariable analysis adjusting for total number of transfusions, age or donor, and birth weight, female donor was associated with a lower risk of the primary outcome (relative risk 0.29; 95% CI 0.16–0.54). The association was modified by the age of the donor (closer to null as donor age decreased).

(continued on next page)

Table 1
(continued)

First Author[ref] (Year of Publication)	Type of Study	Population (Sample Size)	Unit of Analysis (Infant or RBC Transfusion Episode)	Primary Comparison	Primary Outcome	Summary of Main Findings
Murphy et al,[34] 2018	Observational cohort study (retrospective)	Preterm infants <32 wk gestation (n = 170)	Infant	Infants receiving RBCs from any female donors (±male donor), compared with exclusively male donors.	BPD, any major morbidity (death, BPD, IVH, PVL, ROP, SIP, NEC)	In analyses adjusted for the number of transfusions, receipt of any female donor blood was not associated with BPD (OR 1.44; 95% CI 0.64–3.25), any major morbidity (OR 1.50; 95% CI 0.65–3.45) or length of stay (mean difference 4.8 d, P = .46).

All studies identified from a systematic search strategy were included in this table.
Abbreviations: BPD, bronchopulmonary dysplasia; CI, confidence interval; IL, interleukin; IVH, intraventricular hemorrhage; NEC, necrotizing enterocolitis; PVL, periventricular leukomalacia; RBC, red blood cell; ROP, retinopathy of prematurity; SIP, spontaneous intestinal perforation; TNF, tumor necrosis factor; VLBW, very low birth weight.

BLOOD DONOR SEX AND VERY LOW BIRTH WEIGHT INFANT MORBIDITY AND MORTALITY

Three studies have evaluated the association between blood donor sex and death or serious morbidity in VLBW infants (see **Table 1**). Murphy and colleagues[34] studied 462 infants less than 32 weeks gestation at Woman and Infants Hospital in Rhode Island from 2009 to 2010. Among these infants, 190 received RBC transfusion and infants who received only male donor blood were compared with those who received female donor blood (may have also received male donor blood). Infants who also received platelet or plasma transfusion ($N = 20$) were excluded. The hospital used dedicated donor units, so individual units were assigned to a specific infant until the unit either expired or had an insufficient volume for transfusion. RBC transfusion was prepared by gravity sedimentation centrifugation to a hematocrit of 55% to 65% and stored in citrate phosphate double dextrose and RBCs were not centrifuged before transfusion. In unadjusted analyses, the study reported that infants who received female blood ($\pm$ male blood), compared with only male donor blood, had higher rates of BPD (38% vs 22%, $P = .03$), NEC or spontaneous intestinal perforation (17% vs 6%, $P = .04$) and death or any morbidity (60% vs 38%, $P = 0.006$). In addition, infants who received female donor blood ($\pm$ male blood), compared with only male donor blood, had a 3 week longer hospitalization ($P = .01$). However, when adjusted for the total number of transfusions, there was no significant associations with outcomes ($P = .38$ for BPD, $P = .34$ for any major morbidity and $P = .46$ for length of stay). In addition, the study reported an interaction between female donor blood ($\pm$ male blood), compared with only male donor blood, and number of transfusions on any major morbidity ($P = .015$), suggesting that the association between transfusions and morbidity may potentially depend on the sex of the blood donor. In this analysis, the number of transfusions was similar between infants receiving female donor blood versus male donor blood (mean $\pm$ SD of 3.0 $\pm$ 3 vs 3.4 $\pm$ 3 respectively, $P = .28$), although the number of transfusions was associated with each of the outcomes ($P = .01$ for BPD, $P = .04$ for any major morbidity, and $P = .007$ for length of stay). The investigators acknowledged that the analysis did not consider the timing of transfusion in relation to the diagnosis of the outcomes of interest, such that causation could not be determined.

Patel and colleagues[33] performed a secondary analysis of a prospective cohort study of VLBW infants who were enrolled at three Atlanta, Georgia hospitals from 2010 to 2014. Out of 598 infants, 343 received RBC transfusion and 324 had donor and covariate data available for analysis. Of these 324 infants, 143 received RBC transfusions from both male and female donors and were excluded. This was done because of the inability to assign a single consistent donor sex exposure. The remaining 181 infants who received 499 transfusions were studied. Blood donor sex information was not recorded on the blood units and not available to the blood bank personnel as part of routine practice or used to decide allocation of units. The RBCs transfused were O-negative, cytomegalovirus seronegative, irradiated, leukocyte reduced, and stored in citrate phosphate dextrose adenine (CPDA-1) solution. Similar to the blood banking practices in the prior study by Murphy and colleagues.[34], study centers used dedicated single-donor units for each infant to minimize donor exposure for neonatal transfusion.

The study reported that VLBW infants receiving RBC transfusion from only female donors, compared with only males, had a lower risk of death or serious morbidity (BPD, NEC, and ROP). Infants receiving RBC transfusions from only female donors had a 21% risk of a serious adverse composite outcome, compared with 45% of infants receiving transfusions from only male donors, corresponding to an absolute risk difference of 23%. This protective association between RBC transfusions from female donors, compared with male donors, and a lower risk of a serious adverse composite outcome increased as the donor age increased (interaction $P = .005$). For the typical infant, who received a median of two transfusions, RBC transfusion from exclusively female donors, compared with male donors, was associated with a lower risk of the primary outcome in multivariable analyses (adjusted relative risk, 0.29; 95% CI, 0.16–0.54). The median number of RBC transfusions was similar between male and female donors (two transfusions). In addition, estimates of individual components, except for ROP, were consistent in direction with the major components of the composite outcome (Fig. 2). Similar findings were found in analysis limited to infants receiving only one RBC transfusion and in analyses that accounted for gestational age, storage age of RBCs, storage age following irradiation, multiple donor exposure, illness severity scores, and center. The study did not consider additional donor characteristics such as smoking, pregnancy status, or medication use, as these were considered to be part of the effect of donor sex. The investigators concluded that additional confirmatory and mechanistic studies to evaluate the impact of blood donor sex were warranted.

More recently, Bahr and colleagues[31] evaluated a cohort of all neonates receiving at least one RBC transfusion during a 12-year period from 2009 to 2021 from 15 Intermountain Healthcare hospitals. Among a cohort of 2086 infants, 825 infants received RBCs from exclusively female donors, 935 infants were transfused exclusively with RBCs from male donors, and 326 infants were transfused with RBCs from both female and male donors. The transfused units were irradiated, leukoreduced, and stored in CPDA-1 solution. The association between a composite outcome of death or moderate/severe BPD, moderate/severe NEC, or severe ROP was evaluated with adjustment for birth weight, number of transfusions, and sex of the recipient, with account for clustering by hospital. There was no association between the primary outcome for infants who received RBCs from only male donors versus only female donors (52% vs 49%; adjusted relative risk (RR): 1.05; 95% CI 0.92–1.20; $P = .47$). Similar findings were noted for components of the composite outcome. In addition, there were no significant differences based on recipient sex or donor age.

Taken together, these three studies report conflicting findings, with two studies[31,34] reporting no association between blood donor sex and mortality or serious morbidity in adjusted analyses and one[33] reporting protective association in which infants transfused with RBCs from female donors had a lower risk of death or serious morbidity. Of note, both the study by Murphy and colleagues[34] and Patel and colleagues[33] reported an interaction between the number of RBC transfusions and outcomes, suggesting

	Risk of infant outcome by donor exposure, n/N (%)		Adjusted odds ratio (95% CI)	Favors female RBC donor	Favors male RBC donor
	Female donor	Male donor			
Composite	12/56 (21.4%)	56/125 (44.8%)	0.26 (0.09-0.65)		
BPD	9/56 (16.1%)	35/125 (28.0%)	0.52 (0.18-1.35)		
Death	2/56 (3.6%)	15/125 (12.0%)	0.27 (0.03-1.29)		
NEC	1/56 (1.8%)	12/125 (9.6%)	0.17 (0.004-1.19)		
ROP	1/56 (1.8%)	3/125 (2.4%)	1.00 (0.02-18.33)		

0.01   0.1   1   10
Odds ratio (95% CI)

Fig. 2. Outcomes in transfused VLBW infants by blood donor sex. Estimates include adjustment for total number transfusions, birth weight, and donor age. BPD, bronchopulmonary dysplasia; NEC, necrotizing enterocolitis; ROP, retinopathy of prematurity. (*Figure reproduced from* Patel et al.[33] with open access CC-BY license.)

that donor sex may modify this relationship. In both studies, the number of RBC transfusions was similar between donor sex groups, suggesting that this was not a major confounder. Because units are not allocated for transfusion based on the sex of the donor, confounding by indication is unlikely to bias findings. However, it is important to note that blood donors may be in close geographic proximity to blood suppliers, and each of these three studies included hospitals in different geographic regions of the United States. In the next two sections, the authors review studies examining the effects of blood donor sex on changes in pro-inflammatory cytokines around transfusion and on transfusion effectiveness measured by increases in hemoglobin increment following RBC transfusion.

BLOOD DONOR SEX AND TRANSFUSION-MEDIATED INFLAMMATION IN PRETERM INFANTS

Prior studies have reported that RBC transfusions are associated with increases in pro-inflammatory cytokine expression and endothelial activation in preterm infants.[2,3,36] In a secondary analysis of a prior study,[36] changes in cytokine concentrations were compared from before to after RBC transfusion by both donor sex and if the RBCs were washed or unwashed. The study found that unwashed RBC transfusions from female donors were associated with increases in pro-inflammatory cytokines, and this was reduced with washing of RBCs. The changes in cytokines were most pronounced with the third RBC transfusion, suggesting the potential impact of repeated exposures to RBC transfusion, and were different for interleukin (IL)-6 ($P = .003$), IL-12 ($P = .008$), IL-17A ($P = .003$), and tumor necrosis factor (TNF) ($P = .007$). Washing lowered levels of IL-6, IL-12, and TNF associated with RBC transfusions from female donors. The investigators noted that RBC transfusion results in exposure of neonates and infants to potentially immunomodulatory factors that might impact white blood cell (WBC) priming, neutrophil chemotaxis, monocyte/macrophage activation and cytokine production,[37] potentially from WBC-derived mediators, free heme, and microparticles.[38] However, the mechanistic basis for why RBC transfusions are pro-inflammatory in preterm infants is still uncertain.

BLOOD DONOR SEX AND TRANSFUSION EFFECTIVENESS

In a study by DeSimone and colleagues,[30] a linked vein-to-vein database was used to evaluate donor and component factors associated with RBC transfusion effectiveness in VLBW infants, measured based on posttransfusion hemoglobin increments. The study used the National Heart, Lung, and Blood Institute Recipient Epidemiology and Donor Evaluation Study III cohort, which included infants cared for at seven academic and community hospitals in the United States from 2013 to 2016. Changes in hemoglobin increments from the 24 hours before RBC transfusion to the hemoglobin measure closest to the end of RBC transfusion (within 24 hours) were calculated and associated factors were evaluated using multivariable regression. Of the 254 VLBW infants included, 567 RBC transfusion episodes were studied. The mean (±SD) hemoglobin increment following RBC transfusion was 1.9 g/dL ± 2.1. Female donor sex (−0.24 g/dL; 95% CI −0.02, −0.57), donor age less than 25 years (−0.57 g/dL; 95% CI − 1.02, −0.11), male recipient sex (−0.36 g/dL; 95% CI −0.35, −1.50), higher pretransfusion hemoglobin levels (−0.70 g/dL; 95% CI −0.79, −0.61), and concomitant plasma transfusion (−0.64 g/dL; 95% CI −−1.06, −0.23) were each independently associated with decreased posttransfusion hemoglobin increments in VLBW infants. Among infants receiving RBC transfusion from male donors, the odds of a subsequent transfusion event within 48 hours were greater (odds ratio 3.0; 95% CI 1.3, 6.7) if donors had hemoglobin less than 13.5 g/dL. This study supports the premise that blood donor characteristics can influence the effectiveness of RBC transfusion in VLBW infants.

ADDITIONAL CONSIDERATIONS RELATED TO BLOOD DONOR SEX

There are many factors that may result in differences in donor RBC units obtained from males, compared with females, with some attributed to biological differences, and other differences potentially related to behaviors, lifestyle, health conditions, disease, and blood bank factors that might be associated with sex and gender (**Fig. 3**). Although this is not a primary focus of this review, the authors briefly discuss these additional donor characteristics below.

Female RBCs are noted to have lower hemoglobin, are younger, more deformable and less fragile during storage, and have increased oxygen carrying capacity.[39–42] Some of these differences are due to the loss of RBCs from menstruation in females. As previously discussed, these factors may explain the reduced posttransfusion hemoglobin increments observed from female donors in VLBW infants,[30] similar to findings in adult recipients.[43]

Beyond biological differences, additional considerations include potential differences between males and females in behavior, lifestyle, and health conditions that might also contribute to differences in RBC donation quality. Although these factors are complex and not always associated with sex or gender, there is a potential impact of the blood donor exposome as it relates to diet,[44,45] smoking and nicotine exposure,[46,47] alcohol consumption,[48] caffeine intake,[49] iron supplementation,[50] prior pregnancy,[24] diseases such as diabetes,[51] G6PD deficiency,[52] medications,[53] and age of blood donors.[54] Therefore, when considering the impact of the sex of blood donors, the potential mechanisms for the impact on recipient outcomes may involve more than simply sex-related biological differences in RBCs.

Blood banking and donor center practices that might differ by sex include donation intensity,[55] which is associated with iron loss in the donors and the quality of stored RBCs. The potential influence of donor sex on recipient outcomes has been recognized with plasma transfusion and risk of transfusion-related acute lung-injury from female donor plasma.[42] This is mediated by human leukocyte antigen and granulocyte antibodies, which are present in female donors. In addition, RBC antibodies are more common among pregnant donors[56] and could mediate adverse effects in transfused recipients if undetected by antibody screening. Furthermore, donor deferral is more common among male donors.[57] Finally, selection of donors based on factors such as cytomegalovirus (CMV) seropositivity could influence both the age and sex of the blood donor, given CMV seroprevalence increases with age and is more common among females, compared with males.[58] Unique to neonates is the common practice of repeated transfusions from the same donor,[59] which then repeatedly exposes neonates and infants who receive greater than one RBC transfusion from the same donor (including their specific characteristics). Although this practice is not associated with increased alloimmunization, it could expose infants repetitively to either favorable or unfavorable donor characteristics depending on the unit allocated to them in the blood bank. Furthermore, such approaches might be influenced by when blood banks expire units, which could limit the number of potential repeat donor exposures.

LIMITATIONS OF STUDIES TO DATE

There are inherent limitations in observational studies related to donor factors. Although blood banks do not select RBC units for transfusion into neonates based

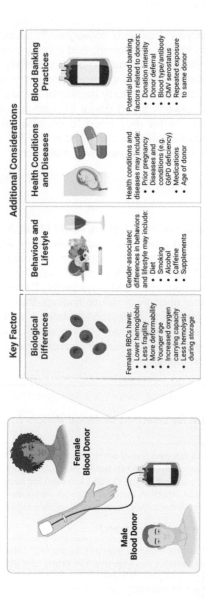

Fig. 3. Potential sex differences in male and female blood donors. CMV, cytomegalovirus; G6PD, glucose-6-phosphate dehydrogenase. (Created with BioRender.com.)

on the sex or age of the donor, there is the potential for bias and confounding due to the interrelated factors between donor sex and transfusion effectiveness impacting the need for subsequent transfusion (treatment-confounder feedback). Accounting for these factors is important as they could bias the association between donor sex and recipient outcomes.[60] Importantly, although blood donor sex is often randomly allocated (unless there is selection on a factor associated with sex, such as CMV sero-negative units), the impact of differences in donors on subsequent need for transfusion could bias findings. In a study by Zhao and colleagues,[60] accounting for treatment-confounder feedback using cloning, censoring, and inverse probability weighting in an approach identical to a marginal structural model, the study found no difference in mortality risk for adult patients undergoing transfusions from female or parous donors, compared with male donors. This study highlights the analytical complexity in assessing the associations between blood donor characteristics and recipient outcomes. Future observational studies may need to consider treatment-confounder feedback, although in the studies to date, the number of RBC transfusions did not meaningfully differ between infants transfused with male donor versus female donor units.

SUMMARY

Emerging literature on the potential impact of the sex of blood donors on outcomes in transfused neonates and infants reports conflicting findings. Additional studies are needed to address this uncertainty, including both epidemiologic studies and mechanistic studies evaluating relevant factors that could explain if there is an impact of blood donor sex on neonatal outcomes and physiology. These studies may provide additional information to either support or refute findings from current observational studies, which would be important to establish before clinical trials of donor-selected RBC transfusion are pursued, as has been recently done in adults.[61] Beyond donor sex, additional studies into *what* is being transfused may guide future improvements in neonatal transfusion therapy.

Best Practices Box

What is the current practice for selection of blood donors for neonatal RBC transfusion?

Currently, blood donors are not selected based on their sex or age for neonatal RBC transfusion. However, blood donors are selected based on routine donor screening questionnaires, their blood type (typically type O RBCs are used for neonatal transfusion) and, sometimes, their cytomegalovirus infection serostatus (some clinicians or centers request transfusion from blood obtained from only cytomegalovirus seronegative donors).

Best practice/guideline/care path objective(s)

What changes in current practice are likely to improve outcomes? Selecting blood donors based on their individual characteristics can improve the safety and efficacy of blood transfusion. However, there is currently insufficient evidence to support the selection of blood donors based on their sex for use in neonatal transfusion.

Major Recommendations

- Future research should evaluate if selection of blood donors based on sex (or other characteristics) can improve outcomes in transfused neonatal recipients. However, unless future research shows a beneficial potential impact of such a strategy on clinical outcomes, current approaches of using RBCs from donors of either sex are recommended.

Bibliographic Source(s)

• Patel RM, Meyer EK, Widness JA. Research opportunities to improve neonatal red blood cell transfusion. Transfus Med Rev. 2016;30(4):165-173. doi:10.1016/j.tmrv.2016.06.005.

ACKNOWLEDGMENTS

The authors would like to acknowledge Shenita Peterson, Systematic Review Coordinator and Public Health Informationist, at Emory University with assistance in the search strategy and identification of articles.

DISCLOSURES

R.M. Patel serves as a consultant for Noveome, Inc and serves on the data-safety monitoring committee for Infant Bacterial Therapeutics/Premier research.

REFERENCES

1. Patel RM, Hendrickson JE, Nellis ME, et al. Variation in neonatal transfusion practice. J Pediatr 2021;235:92–9.e4.
2. Benavides A, Bell EF, Georgieff MK, et al. Sex-specific cytokine responses and neurocognitive outcome after blood transfusions in preterm infants. Pediatr Res 2022;91(4):947–54.
3. Keir AK, McPhee AJ, Andersen CC, et al. Plasma cytokines and markers of endothelial activation increase after packed red blood cell transfusion in the preterm infant. Pediatr Res 2013;73(1):75–9.
4. Ho TTB, Groer MW, Luciano AA, et al. Red blood cell transfusions increase fecal calprotectin levels in premature infants. J Perinatol 2015;35(10):837–41.
5. Guo Y, Wang Y, Marin T, et al. Statistical methods for characterizing transfusion-related changes in regional oxygenation using near-infrared spectroscopy (NIRS) in preterm infants. Stat Methods Med Res 2019;28(9):2710–23.
6. Kalteren WS, Verhagen EA, Mintzer JP, et al. Anemia and red blood cell transfusions, cerebral oxygenation, brain injury and development, and neurodevelopmental outcome in preterm infants: a systematic review. Front Pediatr 2021;9: 644462.
7. Saito-Benz M, Murphy WG, Tzeng Y-C, et al. Storage after gamma irradiation affects in vivo oxygen delivery capacity of transfused red blood cells in preterm infants. Transfusion 2018;58(9):2108–12.
8. Patel RM, Knezevic A, Yang J, et al. Enteral iron supplementation, red blood cell transfusion, and risk of bronchopulmonary dysplasia in very-low-birth-weight infants. Transfusion 2019;59(5):1675–82.
9. Bolat F, Dursun M, Sarıaydın M. Packed red blood cell transfusion as a predictor of moderate-severe bronchopulmonary dysplasia: a comparative cohort study of very preterm infants. Am J Perinatol 2023. https://doi.org/10.1055/a-2051-8245.
10. Zhang Z, Huang X, Lu H. Association between red blood cell transfusion and bronchopulmonary dysplasia in preterm infants. Sci Rep 2014;4:4340.
11. Kalteren WS, Bos AF, Bergman KA, et al. The short-term effects of RBC transfusions on intestinal injury in preterm infants. Pediatr Res 2023;93(5):1307–13.
12. MohanKumar K, Namachivayam K, Song T, et al. A murine neonatal model of necrotizing enterocolitis caused by anemia and red blood cell transfusions. Nat Commun 2019;10(1):3494.

13. Song J, Dong H, Xu F, et al. The association of severe anemia, red blood cell transfusion and necrotizing enterocolitis in neonates. PLoS ONE 2021;16(7). e0254810.
14. Lust C, Vesoulis Z, Jackups R, et al. Early red cell transfusion is associated with development of severe retinopathy of prematurity. J Perinatol 2019;39(3): 393–400.
15. Schecter LV, Medina AE, Alexander JL, et al. Impact of early postnatal exposure of red blood cell transfusions on the severity of retinopathy of prematurity. J Neonatal Perinatal Med 2021;14(4):527–35.
16. Kirpalani H, Bell EF, Hintz SR, et al. Higher or lower hemoglobin transfusion thresholds for preterm infants. N Engl J Med 2020;383(27):2639–51.
17. Franz AR, Engel C, Bassler D, et al. Effects of liberal vs restrictive transfusion thresholds on survival and neurocognitive outcomes in extremely low-birth-weight infants: the ETTNO randomized clinical trial. JAMA 2020;324(6):560–70.
18. Kirpalani H, Whyte RK, Andersen C, et al. The Premature Infants in Need of Transfusion (PINT) study: a randomized, controlled trial of a restrictive (low) versus liberal (high) transfusion threshold for extremely low birth weight infants. J Pediatr 2006;149(3):301–7.
19. Bell EF, Strauss RG, Widness JA, et al. Randomized trial of liberal versus restrictive guidelines for red blood cell transfusion in preterm infants. Pediatrics 2005; 115(6):1685–91.
20. Bell EF. Red cell transfusion thresholds for preterm infants: finally some answers. Arch Dis Child Fetal Neonatal Ed 2022;107(2):126–30.
21. Patel RM, Meyer EK, Widness JA. Research opportunities to improve neonatal red blood cell transfusion. Transfus Med Rev 2016;30(4):165–73.
22. Nilsson AK, Hellgren G, Sjöbom U, et al. Preterm infant circulating sex steroid levels are not altered by transfusion with adult male plasma: a retrospective multi-centre cohort study. Arch Dis Child Fetal Neonatal Ed 2022;107(6):577–82.
23. Karafin MS, Westlake M, Hauser RG, et al. Risk factors for red blood cell alloimmunization in the Recipient Epidemiology and Donor Evaluation Study (REDS-III) database. Br J Haematol 2018;181(5):672–81.
24. Caram-Deelder C, Kreuger AL, Evers D, et al. Association of blood transfusion from female donors with and without a history of pregnancy with mortality among male and female transfusion recipients. JAMA 2017;318(15):1471–8.
25. Middelburg RA, Briët E, van der Bom JG. Mortality after transfusions, relation to donor sex. Vox Sang 2011;101(3):221–9.
26. Kulharya AS, Salbert BA, Norris KN, et al. Packed red cell transfusion does not compromise chromosome analysis in newborns. Genet Med 2001;3(4):314–7.
27. Viëtor HE, Hallensleben E, van Bree SP, et al. Survival of donor cells 25 years after intrauterine transfusion. Blood 2000;95(8):2709–14.
28. Romano M, el Marsafy A, Marseglia GL, et al. Increased percentage of activated Ia+ T lymphocytes in peripheral blood of neonates following exchange blood transfusion. Clin Immunol Immunopathol 1987;43(3):301–7.
29. Sacks MS, Spurling CL, Bross IDJ, et al. Study of the influence of sex of donor on the survival of erythroblastotic infants treated by exchange transfusion. Pediatrics 1950;6(5):772–7.
30. DeSimone RA, Plimier C, Goel R, et al. Associations of donor, component, and recipient factors on hemoglobin increments following red blood cell transfusion in very low birth weight infants. Transfusion 2023. https://doi.org/10.1111/trf. 17468.

31. Bahr TM, Christensen TR, Tweddell SM, et al. Associations between blood donor sex and age, and outcomes of transfused newborn infants. Transfusion 2023. https://doi.org/10.1111/trf.17417.

32. Crawford T, Andersen C, Marks DC, et al. Does donor sex influence the potential for transfusion with washed packed red blood cells to limit transfusion-related immune responses in preterm newborns? Arch Dis Child Fetal Neonatal Ed 2023. https://doi.org/10.1136/archdischild-2022-324531.

33. Patel RM, Lukemire J, Shenvi N, et al. Association of blood donor sex and age with outcomes in very low-birth-weight infants receiving blood transfusion. JAMA Netw Open 2021;4(9). e2123942.

34. Murphy T, Chawla A, Tucker R, et al. Impact of blood donor sex on transfusion-related outcomes in preterm infants. J Pediatr 2018;201:215–20.

35. Crawford TM, Andersen CC, Stark MJ. Red blood cell donor sex associated effects on morbidity and mortality in the extremely preterm newborn. Children (Basel). 2022;9(12).

36. Crawford TM, Andersen CC, Hodyl NA, et al. Effect of washed versus unwashed red blood cells on transfusion-related immune responses in preterm newborns. Clin Transl Immunol 2022;11(3):e1377.

37. Muszynski JA, Spinella PC, Cholette JM, et al. Transfusion-related immunomodulation: review of the literature and implications for pediatric critical illness. Transfusion 2017;57(1):195–206.

38. Remy KE, Hall MW, Cholette J, et al. Mechanisms of red blood cell transfusion-related immunomodulation. Transfusion 2018;58(3):804–15.

39. Mykhailova O, Olafson C, Turner TR, et al. Donor-dependent aging of young and old red blood cell subpopulations: metabolic and functional heterogeneity. Transfusion 2020;60(11):2633–46.

40. Kameneva MV, Watach MJ, Borovetz HS. Gender difference in rheologic properties of blood and risk of cardiovascular diseases. Clin Hemorheol Microcirc 1999; 21(3–4):357–63.

41. Kanias T, Lanteri MC, Page GP, et al. Ethnicity, sex, and age are determinants of red blood cell storage and stress hemolysis: results of the REDS-III RBC-Omics study. Blood Adv 2017;1(15):1132–41.

42. Ning S, Heddle NM, Acker JP. Exploring donor and product factors and their impact on red cell post-transfusion outcomes. Transfus Med Rev 2018;32(1): 28–35.

43. Roubinian NH, Plimier C, Woo JP, et al. Effect of donor, component, and recipient characteristics on hemoglobin increments following red blood cell transfusion. Blood 2019;134(13):1003–13.

44. Unruh D, Srinivasan R, Benson T, et al. Red blood cell dysfunction induced by high-fat diet: potential implications for obesity-related atherosclerosis. Circulation 2015;132(20):1898–908.

45. Benson TW, Weintraub NL, Kim HW, et al. A single high-fat meal provokes pathological erythrocyte remodeling and increases myeloperoxidase levels: implications for acute coronary syndrome. Lab Invest 2018;98(10):1300–10.

46. Stefanoni D, Fu X, Reisz JA, et al. Nicotine exposure increases markers of oxidant stress in stored red blood cells from healthy donor volunteers. Transfusion 2020; 60(6):1160–74.

47. DeSimone RA, Hayden JA, Mazur CA, et al. Red blood cells donated by smokers: a pilot investigation of recipient transfusion outcomes. Transfusion 2019;59(8): 2537–43.

48. D'Alessandro A, Fu X, Reisz JA, et al. Ethyl glucuronide, a marker of alcohol consumption, correlates with metabolic markers of oxidant stress but not with hemolysis in stored red blood cells from healthy blood donors. Transfusion 2020;60(6): 1183–96.

49. D'Alessandro A, Fu X, Reisz JA, et al. Stored RBC metabolism as a function of caffeine levels. Transfusion 2020;60(6):1197–211.

50. Crowder LA, Cable RG, Spencer BR. Validity of donor-reported iron supplementation practices obtained at the time of donation. Transfusion 2023;63(3):470–5.

51. Li H, Fang K, Peng H, et al. The relationship between glycosylated hemoglobin level and red blood cell storage lesion in blood donors. Transfusion 2022;62(3): 663–74.

52. Roubinian NH, Reese SE, Qiao H, et al. Donor genetic and nongenetic factors affecting red blood cell transfusion effectiveness. JCI Insight 2022;7(1).

53. Nemkov T, Stefanoni D, Bordbar A, et al. Blood donor exposome and impact of common drugs on red blood cell metabolism. JCI Insight 2021;6(3).

54. Cloutier M, Cognasse F, Yokoyama APH, et al. Quality assessment of red blood cell concentrates from blood donors at the extremes of the age spectrum: the BEST collaborative study. Transfusion 2023.

55. Kanias T, Stone M, Page GP, et al. Frequent blood donations alter susceptibility of red blood cells to storage- and stress-induced hemolysis. Transfusion 2019; 59(1):67–78.

56. Karafin MS, Tan S, Tormey CA, et al. Prevalence and risk factors for RBC alloantibodies in blood donors in the recipient Epidemiology and donor evaluation study-III (REDS-III). Transfusion 2019;59(1):217–25.

57. Lamba DS, Sachdev S, Hans R, et al. Review of blood donor deferral with emphasis on donor and patient safety. Transfus Clin Biol 2023;30(1):56–62.

58. van Boven M, van de Kassteele J, Korndewal MJ, et al. Infectious reactivation of cytomegalovirus explaining age- and sex-specific patterns of seroprevalence. Plos Comput Biol 2017;13(9). e1005719.

59. Strauss RG, Johnson K, Cress G, et al. Alloimmunization in preterm infants after repeated transfusions of WBC-reduced RBCs from the same donor. Transfusion 2000;40(12):1463–8.

60. Zhao J, Sjölander A, Edgren G. Mortality among patients undergoing blood transfusion in relation to donor sex and parity: a natural experiment. JAMA Intern Med 2022;182(7):747–56.

61. Chassé M, Fergusson DA, Tinmouth A, et al. Effect of donor sex on recipient mortality in transfusion. N Engl J Med 2023;388(15):1386–95.

Neonatal Blood Banking Practices

Elizabeth P. Crowe, MD, PhD[a], Ruchika Goel, MD, MPH[b,c,d],
Nour Al-Mozain, MD[e,f], Cassandra D. Josephson, MD[g,h],*

KEYWORDS

- Neonate • Premature • Red blood cells • Platelets • Transfusion

KEY POINTS

- Blood bank testing workflows uniquely omit the initial reverse blood type plasma testing for anti-A and anti-B along with repeat ABO/RhD and compatibility testing for neonates (<4 months) when specific criteria are met.
- The direct antiglobulin test is useful in the evaluation of clinically suspected immune-mediated hemolysis such as in a transfusion reaction workup or investigation of hemolytic disease of the newborn, but functions poorly as a screening test.
- Neonates warrant special consideration when selecting blood components for transfusion due to their small total blood volumes and susceptibility to volume overload and metabolic derangements.
- Special populations and transfusion scenarios such as fresh whole blood for congenital heart disease surgery, use of reconstituted whole blood for neonatal exchange transfusion, and transfusion support for ABO-incompatible heart transplants in neonates are discussed.

INTRODUCTION

Neonatologists and transfusion medicine experts differ in their definitions of a neonate. The clinical definition refers to a child less than 28 day old, whereas the blood

[a] Department of Pathology, Johns Hopkins University School of Medicine, 1800 Orleans Street, Sheikh Zayed Tower, Room 3081-A, Baltimore, MD 21287, USA; [b] Corporate Medical Affairs, Vitalant National Office, Scottsdale, AZ, USA; [c] Division of Hematology/Oncology, Department of Internal Medicine and Pediatrics, Simmons Cancer Institute at SIU School of Medicine, 704 Lismore Lane, Springfield, IL 62704, USA; [d] Department of Pathology, Johns Hopkins University School of Medicine, Baltimore, MD, USA; [e] Hematopathology & Transfusion Medicine, Department of Pathology & Laboratory Medicine, King Faisal Specialist Hospital & Research Centre, 7652, Riyadh, Riyadh, 12713, Saudi Arabia; [f] Department of Pathology, College of Medicine, King Saud University, Riyadh, Saudi Arabia; [g] Department of Oncology and Pediatrics, Johns Hopkins University School of Medicine, Baltimore, MD, USA; [h] Cancer and Blood Disorders Institute, Blood Bank and Transfusion Medicine, Department of Pathology, Johns Hopkins All Children's Hospital, St. Petersburg, FL, USA
* Corresponding author. 601 5th Street South, St. Petersburg, FL 33701.
E-mail address: cjosep22@jhmi.edu

Clin Perinatol 50 (2023) 821–837
https://doi.org/10.1016/j.clp.2023.07.008
0095-5108/23/© 2023 Elsevier Inc. All rights reserved.

perinatology.theclinics.com

bank defines a neonate as a child less than 4 months (<120 days) after birth.[1] This discrepancy arises partly due to the peculiarities of Association for the Advancement of Blood & Biotherapies (AABB) Standards as well as the unique immunologic environment in neonates (see "Blood Bank Testing Practices").[2,3]

Neonatal blood banking practices differ from those for other patient groups, and there is limited formal guidance for selecting and processing blood components.[4,5] In addition, significant physiologic heterogeneity exists among neonates, including subpopulations such as preterm infants and those receiving respiratory support or exchange transfusion, each with specific requirements. Even when applying high-quality evidence to blood banking practices, it is crucial to exercise caution, particularly when the study population differs substantially from the actual patients. However, multicenter studies conducted in countries with centralized transfusion services and presumably more standardized practices may yield more generalizable evidence.

BLOOD BANK TESTING PRACTICES
How Is Blood Bank Testing for Neonates Unique?

Pretransfusion testing in neonates is unique due to the physiologic differences in the immune system and red cell immunohematology features from older populations.

Need for a Second Specimen

Neonates are particularly vulnerable to mislabeling or wrong blood in tube (WBIT) errors: this may be due to unique naming conventions (eg, first name "Baby") or confusion with twins and/or a maternal specimen at birth hospitals.[6] Therefore, the two-specimen rule should ideally be applied as a verification method to maintain patient safety unless an electronic patient identification system is in place.[7]

Specimen Source and Collection

Umbilical cord blood, neonatal venous blood, or capillary (heel stick) blood are the primary specimen sources for neonatal blood bank testing. Umbilical cord blood testing minimizes the need for neonatal venipuncture; however, there are concerns about potential contamination with maternal blood or Wharton's jelly, and limited guidelines exist to direct testing practice.[8] In some cases, when available at a birth hospital, maternal plasma/serum may be used to detect unexpected red blood cell (RBC) alloantibodies to preserve the neonatal specimen. To prevent errors such as WBIT, which can lead to misdiagnosis and fatal outcomes, strict adherence to proper specimen collection and labeling technique is crucial.[3]

Routine Blood Bank Tests

The standard testing includes "forward typing" which includes ABO and RhD phenotyping of the neonatal RBCs only. Weak ABO antigen expression in neonates can arise due to different reasons such as mixed-field agglutination after group O transfusion to an A, B, or AB recipient, chimerism, fetomaternal exchange, or inheritance of unusual alleles resulting in weak A/B antigen expression.[9] Results of the "forward testing" should be interpreted cautiously in the setting of prior intrauterine transfusion, as typing may appear as O RhD negative, reflecting the transfused donor blood type. Plasma or serum typing "reverse typing" is not performed because ABO antibodies present in the neonatal plasma after birth are mostly of maternal origin, and the corresponding anti-A and anti-B in the neonatal serum/plasma are usually weak or absent.[10] In circumstances where a non-group O neonate is intended to receive an ABO type-specific blood group, specific red cells that are not compatible with the maternal ABO group, "reverse typing" of the infant should be done.[3]

Antibody screening in the neonatal setting is intended to detect unexpected red cell antibodies, which are mostly of the immunoglobulin G (IgG) isotype and may bind neonatal RBC. Maternal IgG is transported across the placenta by an active, neonatal Fc receptor-mediated process during pregnancy,[11] from approximately 26 weeks of gestation up until birth. They may remain in the circulation of the newborn for up to 26 days and become undetectable by 4 months of life.[12] Therefore, best practice for unexpected antibody detection (antibody screen) is to perform testing on maternal serum/plasma if available; the use of these tests in the neonate should be limited to cases in which a maternal specimen is unavailable.[13]

If the antibody screen is positive or there is a clinical suspicion of immune hemolysis, the direct antiglobulin test (DAT) is performed on the neonatal RBC containing specimen. Although many centers use DAT as a screening test to assess the risk of hemolytic disease in the newborn, it has a poor positive predictive value for the severity of hemolysis and/or the need for phototherapy.[14,15] Therefore, a positive DAT result must be interpreted in the clinical context, along with ancillary laboratory data (eg, bilirubin level and drop in hemoglobin level). Moreover, a negative DAT does not exclude clinically significant hemolysis and it is frequently observed in ABO hemolytic disease of the fetus and newborn,[14] where the recipient is A, B, or AB, and the mother is type O. Despite that an AABB survey performed in Canada and the United States has indicated that around 23% of the participating hospitals mandate DAT testing before discharge.[16]

In transfusion laboratories adopting electronic crossmatch, neonates may be eligible for an electronic crossmatch or are "presumed crossmatch compatible" if the initial antibody screen is negative. Moreover, repeat testing including ABO and RhD typing, may be omitted, and the testing result may be valid for the remainder of the neonate's hospital admission or until the neonate reaches the age of 4 months, whichever is sooner.[3] Of note, the cutoff of 4 months of age for abbreviated blood bank testing was selected based on speculation regarding when maternal antibodies are expected to disappear from neonatal circulation and when neonatal immune function is believed to be competent.[2] However, if the antibody screen is positive, serologic crossmatch is indicated. It is recommended that crossmatching is performed on a maternal specimen, especially for the first transfusion.[13] If a maternal specimen is unavailable and the DAT is positive, it is preferable to use the eluate obtained from the RBC rather than the neonatal serum/plasma for the compatibility testing.[13]

Testing for Evaluation of Fetal and Neonatal Alloimmune Thrombocytopenia

Fetal and neonatal alloimmune thrombocytopenia (FNAIT) is the most common cause of fetal and neonatal severe thrombocytopenia. Noninvasive prenatal testing, available in some centers, using cell-free fetal DNA can determine whether the fetus carries the HPA-1a gene if the biological father is heterozygous for the HPA antigen or unavailable for testing. Chorionic villus sampling is the standard sample source in many centers, but it increases the risk of alloimmunization and fetal loss.[17] The monoclonal antibody immobilization of platelet antigen assay has been widely used to detect alloantibodies in maternal plasma in suspected women.

BLOOD COMPONENT CHARACTERISTICS AND MODIFICATIONS
Donor Characteristics

Blood donor characteristics (eg, age and sex) influence transfusion recipient hemoglobin increments and other outcomes.[18,19] This finding is biologically plausible due to known sex-specific differences impacting RBC rigidity, hemolysis propensity, and antioxidant capacity during storage.[20,21] Transfusions from blood donors of a younger age, those that are sex-mismatched with recipient or from ever-pregnant females have been associated with increased mortality in adult recipients in some studies.[22,23] However, given conflicting observational evidence regarding outcomes with female donors or with sex-mismatched female donors to male recipients, the multicenter, randomized Trial Assessing Donor Sex on Recipient Mortality evaluated survival among adult inpatients who underwent RBC transfusion from primarily male versus primarily female donors (11.4% nonadherence rate); no difference in survival was observed.[24]

Studies of the impact of donor characteristics on recipient outcomes are also relevant to neonates given that transfusion practices favor repeated transfusions from the same donor, thus minimizing donor exposures.[25] Very low birth weight (VLBW) neonates (birth weight ≤1500g and postnatal age ≤5 days) who were transfused RBC from exclusively female blood donors had a lower risk of composite serious morbidity and/or mortality as compared with those that received RBC from exclusively male donors.[25] Furthermore, this beneficial effect of female donors was enhanced with increasing donor age and negated with an increasing number of transfusions on multivariable analysis. By contrast, a separate study in preterm infants (<32 weeks of gestation) failed to identify an association between donor sex and recipient morbidity/mortality after adjusting for the number of RBC transfusions.[26]

An enhanced understanding of the relationship between donor characteristics and recipient outcomes may help to optimize future component selection. In actuality, demographic information about the blood donor is not readily available at the hospital level. Although this information may be obtainable from the blood supplier, it remains clinically inaccessible for routine practice. More information about the impact of blood donors on neonatal outcomes is discussed in another Chapter in this issue.

Post-collection Age of Blood (Freshness)

RBCs incur a storage lesion that impairs oxygen delivery to tissues, yet the overall clinical impact remains unclear.[27] The Age of Red Blood Cells in Premature Infants (ARIPI) trial randomized premature, VLBW (<1250 g) neonates in the NICU to receive "fresh" RBC (mean age 5.1 days) or "standard issue" RBC (mean age 14.6 days).[28] Despite a similar and reportedly liberal transfusion strategy, no difference was observed, as fresh RBCs were not associated with improved outcomes. The generalizability the ARIPI trial was questioned due to (1) lack of specificity and standardization of transfusion thresholds with concerns about applicability to settings with a more restrictive transfusion practice, (2) differences in outcomes related to RBC anticoagulant/additive solution (AS), and (3) differences in storage duration between Canadian and US centers.[29]

Similarly, the Age of Blood in Children in Pediatric Intensive Care Unit (ABC-PICU) study found no difference in organ dysfunction and/or mortality between those transfused with "fresh" RBC (median 5 days) versus "standard issue" RBC (median 18 days) including a subset of neonates (n = 54) who were ≤ 28 days old in the PICU.[30] The volume of RBC transfused per patient was similar between the groups. Of note, the ARIPI and ABC-PICU trials excluded specific patient subsets, including those undergoing cardiac surgery.

The upper limit of RBC storage age for neonates remains uncertain; however, the Food and Drug Administration (FDA) stipulates a maximum allowable storage duration of up to 35 days for units collected in citrate-phosphate-dextrose-adenine (CPDA-1) and 42 days for RBC units collected in AS (eg, AS-1/AS-3).[31] This storage duration is also shortened with irradiation. Although blood banking practices often stipulate a storage threshold for RBC transfused to neonates, they may vary in defining "fresh RBC."[1,32] Balancing the desire for fresher RBC with the preference for minimizing donor exposures continues to be a major challenge for the blood bank.

Component Manufacturing and Processing: Storage Solutions

During collection and processing RBCs are suspended in storage media that enhance RBC viability and prolong storage duration. Typically, RBC units suspended in anticoagulant-preservative solutions such as CPDA-1 have higher hematocrit (65%–80%) compared with those suspended in additive solutions such as AS-1 or AS-3 (hematocrit 55%–65%).[33] ASs extend the storage duration of RBC units reducing the need for frequent donor exposures, but AS exposes the recipient to constituents such as adenine, dextrose, mannitol, and sodium chloride.[4,34]

Given small blood volumes and neonatal vulnerability to metabolic derangements, concerns exist regarding the potential renal toxicity of adenine and the impact of mannitol on cerebral blood flow.[34] Two small prospective, randomized controlled trials (RCT) of small-volume (15 mL/kg/dose) RBC transfusion with AS-1 or AS-3 in premature neonates failed to demonstrate harm; however, these studies were not designed to address the question of harm appropriately.[35,36] Despite widespread use, the safety of large-volume RBC transfusion (>20 mL/kg) containing AS in neonates remains uncertain and large RCTs are lacking for this scenario. The lack of guidance underlies institution-specific practice variability with many blood banks maintaining mixed inventories for specific patient subsets (eg, those requiring exchange transfusion or who are on extracorporeal membrane oxygenation).[1] Furthermore, efforts to limit neonatal RBC transfusion to units collected in CPDA-1 or washing/volume reduction may be unnecessary[37] but is still a common practice in many neonatal units across the US.

Component Manufacturing and Processing: Cytomegalovirus Risk Mitigation

Transfusion–transmission of cytomegalovirus (CMV) is a significant concern for neonatologists due to the potential for devastating, long-term clinical sequelae, especially in the VLBW neonate.[38,39] Historically, rates of CMV transmission via blood transfusion in at-risk recipients were alarmingly high.[40] To mitigate this risk, two main strategies are used by blood suppliers: prestorage leukocyte reduction (LR) and collection of blood components from CMV seronegative donors. The latter strategy does not account for window period donations and greatly restricts the availability of blood as most donors (over 83%) would not qualify based on this criterion, although there is significant geographic variation.[41,42]

LR via filtration effectively removes white blood cells, specifically monocytes, potentially harboring CMV DNA by up to 3 to 4 log 10 (99.9%), but it does not address the cell-free CMV DNA in plasma.[43] Prestorage LR offers other advantages such as a decreased incidence of febrile non-hemolytic transfusion reactions and a lower risk of alloimmunization to human leukocyte antigens (HLA).[44,45]

The phrase "CMV safe" has been extensively adopted for cellular blood products as the primary strategy for preventing transfusion-transmitted CMV[46]; however, the optimal approach for VLBW neonates remains the subject of ongoing debate and practice variability.[1] One contributing factor is the lack of direct comparison studies between a single strategy (either LR or CMV seronegative donors alone) versus an additive combination, referred to as the "belt and suspenders approach."[47] A combined approach completely prevented transmission CMV via transfusion in VLBW neonates (n = 310 receiving 2061 transfusions); however, CMV infection was postnatally acquired in 6.9% of this cohort by 12 weeks of age and largely attributable to maternal breast milk.[48] A follow-up comparative effectiveness pilot study in VLBW neonates (n = 8 receiving 43 transfusions) effectively prevented CMV transfusion–transmission using only LR.[49] In the absence of evidence of superiority for the combination approach, urgent RBC and/or platelet transfusions should not be delayed to provide CMV seronegative components when LR components are readily available.[50] Given how uncommon transfusion-transmitted CMV is in the modern era and the challenges with risk estimation, large comparative trials are unlikely to be feasible. Overall, compared with the risk of CMV transmission via breast milk (reportedly 14.4% [95% CI = 10.1%–20.2%] in a recent meta-analysis of low birth weight or premature infants n = 1920), the risk of transfusion-transmitted CMV is likely very low.[51]

Component Modification: Irradiation

Irradiation of whole blood or cellular blood components (eg, RBC, platelets, granulocytes, or liquid plasma, never frozen) prevents the proliferation of T-lymphocytes that cause transfusion-associated graft versus host disease (TA-GvHD).[52] TA-GvHD is a rare but largely fatal complication of any transfusion containing viable blood donor T-lymphocytes. Generally accepted indications for irradiation include (1) a known or suspected cellular or combined immunodeficiency, (2) significant immune suppression from myelosuppressive chemotherapies or radiation, (3) receipt of intrauterine (ie, RBCs or platelets), or neonatal exchange transfusion, (4) receipt of blood components from HLA matched/compatible blood donors, blood relatives, or any granulocyte transfusion, (5) hematopoietic stem cell transplant recipients/candidates, and (6) hematologic malignancy or Hodgkin lymphoma.[4,5]

An important consideration for rapid and safe provision of irradiated blood components pertains to whether irradiation is performed on-site or whether irradiated components must be obtained from an outside blood supplier and stored as irradiated in the blood bank.[4] To improve efficiency and safety, cesium-based (gamma) blood irradiators are being phased out in favor or x-ray irradiators, which offer higher throughput, faster turnaround time, and reduced susceptibility to biosecurity incidents associated with high-activity radioactive materials.[53]

Although some hospital blood banks practice universal irradiation of cellular blood products up to a specified age to avoid missing an undiagnosed immunodeficiency syndrome, others selectively perform irradiation for specific indications.[1,54] Although preterm neonates are considered at an increased risk of TA-GvHD, due to their relatively immature immune systems, universal irradiation for this patient population is controversial.[4] Irradiation practice for neonates relies on expert opinion and evidence-based guidelines are lacking.

Of note, irradiation can have unintended detrimental effects on component quality and possibly transfusion efficacy, particularly for RBC as documented in numerous studies.[55–57] A recent RCT involving preterm neonates (n = 42, born at less than <34 weeks' gestation and who were at least 14 days old) demonstrated that transfusing freshly irradiated RBC resulted in a slight improvement in cerebral oxygenation compared with transfusing irradiated and stored RBC.[57] This improvement persisted for at least 5 days. Although there are alternatives to irradiation for platelets, such as pathogen inactivation, no approved alternative exists for irradiating RBCs.[58] Irradiation leads to an increase in extracellular potassium in the RBC supernatant, making it crucial to irradiate RBCs close to the time of transfusion to minimize the risk of transfusion-associated hyperkalemia (TAH).[59] Patients who receive high-volume transfusions (>20 mL/kg/dose), such as those requiring a double volume exchange transfusion or requiring transfusion via central venous access with instillation near the right atrium, are at the highest risk of developing cardiac arrhythmias due to TAH.[60]

Component Modification: Washing and Volume Reduction

Washing and volume reduction modifications decrease the volume of plasma and/or AS in a unit of RBCs or platelets. Although there are specific indications for these modifications, they should be considered judiciously due to several drawbacks. These include transfusion delays in obtaining modified components, shorter expiration times (24 hours for RBC and 4 hours for platelets), and decreased yield of RBC and platelets leading to worse transfusion increments.[61–63] The availability of the blood bank to wash or volume reduce cellular blood component neonates varies.

One common indication for washing RBCs is to mitigate TAH in susceptible neonates (see Component Modification: Irradiation).[1] The amount of extracellular potassium in the RBC supernatant depends on factors such as post-collection age, storage duration postirradiation, and the type of storage solution used.[64] Although effective in reducing the immediate concentration of extracellular potassium, washed RBC should ideally be transfused promptly due to increases in extracellular potassium with storage after washing.[59] Other less common indications for washing include recurrent, severe allergic transfusion reactions (eg, IgA deficiency with anti-IgA), and when removal of maternal antibody is need because treatment of the infant with maternal RBCs or platelets is deemed necessary.[1,4] Furthermore, transfusion of washed RBC units is associated with a reduced posttransfusion pro-inflammatory response in preterm neonates.[65]

Volume reduction removes a majority of the incompatible plasma containing anti-A and anti-B isohemagglutinins (IHs). This is performed to minimize the risk of potentially significant passive hemolysis in neonates receiving ABO-incompatible platelet transfusions.[66] Although studies are lacking in neonates, alternatives such as transfusion of platelets in platelet AS (PAS) or units confirmed to have a low titer of incompatible IHs may show promise.[67,68]

Volume reduction may also be indicated to decrease the risk for transfusion-associated circulatory overload (TACO) in susceptible neonates. It is important to consider that centrifugation as part of volume reduction or washing leads to platelet activation with uncertain impact on transfusion outcomes.[69,70] As a result, the practice of concentration of an entire apheresis unit (minimum yield 3×10^{11} platelets suspended in 250–300 mL) into a very small volume for neonatal transfusion should be discouraged.

Component Selection of Red Blood Cells

The practice of selecting only group O RBCs for non-emergent transfusion of neonates regardless of their ABO group remains common.[1,16] This approach eliminates the need for testing of neonatal serum/plasma for passively acquired maternal anti-A, anti-B, or anti-A,B antibodies through the antihuman globulin phase[3]; however, it may place an unnecessary strain on the group O RBC inventory. In one single-center study of neonates ($n = 1309$), only 6.4% had detectable maternal IHs, which were completely cleared from neonatal circulation by the fifth week of life.[12] The decision to pursue group-specific versus group O only RBC transfusion for neonates may differ in birth hospitals as compared with freestanding children's hospitals where maintaining a large inventory of group O RBC may be challenging.

There are limited data regarding outcomes comparing transfusion of group O RBCs to neonatal recipients who are group O versus non-group O. One study of transfused premature neonates in the neonatal intensive care unit (NICU) ($n = 724$) who were either group O (48.8%) or non-group O (51.2%) failed to detect a difference in outcomes such as mortality, length of stay, and other complications.[71] By contrast, another single-center retrospective study of neonates ($n = 276$) in the NICU found group AB infants to be at an increased risk of necrotizing enterocolitis (NEC) (hazard ratio [HR] 2.87; 95% CI 1.40–5.89; P = .003); however, a sub-analysis of AB neonates stratified according to transfusion burden was not possible based the low sample size.[72] In contrast, a recent retrospective multicenter cohort study conducted in VLBW (</ = 1500 g) neonates in the NICU revealed higher all-cause mortality occurred in neonates without NEC who were non-O compared with O (HR = 17.5; 95% CI: 1.78–171.7), but not in neonates with NEC (HR = 1.11; 95% CI: 0.14–8.84). The study suggested ABO nonidentical transfusion was not associated with NEC or mortality in neonates with NEC, although it was associated with increased mortality in neonates without NEC.[73] As many NICUs transfuse only O group blood as routine practice, future trials are needed to investigate the association between this practice and neonatal mortality.

Component Selection of Platelets

Platelets can be prepared from a whole blood donation (usual volume 40–70 mL of plasma, yield $\geq 5.5 \times 10^{10}$ platelets) or collected via apheresis in plasma with or without PAS (usual volume 250–300 mL, $\geq 3.0 \times 10^{11}$ platelets) and prepared as aliquot.[33]

Apheresis platelets that undergo additional processing known as pathogen inactivation to minimize the risk of transfusion-transmitted infections are considered pathogen reduced (PR). The chemical inactivation preventing replication of pathogens also prevents donor T-cell proliferation of the product, negating the need for irradiation of the platelet product. PR platelets have become increasingly prevalent in clinical use despite the increased cost and association with worse increments and increased platelet transfusion burden.[74,75] Of the limited studies of PR platelets that include neonates, none has demonstrated an increased risk of transfusion-related adverse events or clinically significant bleeding as assessed by the surrogate markers of RBC and plasma use.[76–78]

Platelet units that are ABO identical or plasma compatible with the recipient should be selected to minimize the risk of passive hemolysis.[68] If plasma-compatible platelets are unavailable, consider washing and volume reduction (see Component Modification: Washing and Volume Reduction). Moreover, RhD alloimmunization risk from platelet transfusion is exceptionally low, particularly in neonates receiving apheresis products due to little RBC contamination of the product. Therefore, providing RhD positive apheresis platelet transfusion to RhD negative neonatal recipients may be considered appropriate in cases of limited supply.[79] Finally, for neonates with confirmed or suspected FNAIT, if compatible antigen-negative platelets are not readily available, then ABO/Rh compatible antigen-untested platelets may be acceptable.[4,80]

Component Selection of Plasma and Cryoprecipitate

Plasma is a source of pro- and anticoagulant factors that is stored frozen and must be thawed before use. Although most neonatal blood banks select plasma components that are ABO identical or compatible to the neonate for nonurgent transfusions, some centers only transfuse "universal plasma" (ie, group AB) to neonates regardless of transfusion urgency or recipient ABO group.[1] Given that group AB donors comprise up to 4% of all blood donors, this "universal plasma" can be difficult to obtain; therefore, a single unit of AB plasma may be assigned to several neonates. Solvent detergent (SD) plasma is a pathogen-inactivated pooled preparation of plasma that is increasingly used due to myriad benefits. SD plasma is considered safe and is associated with a reduced risk of allergic transfusion reactions, transfusion-related acute lung injury, and possible improved survival.[81–83]

Cryoprecipitate (cryoprecipitated antihemophilic factor or "cryo") is the primary source of fibrinogen replacement with a minimum of 150 mg of fibrinogen per single donor unit in a variable volume (approximately 10–15 mL).[33] Similar to plasma, cryoprecipitate contains anti-A and anti-B IHs. Although ABO-incompatible cryoprecipitate transfusion may be considered a safe and acceptable practice in adults, ABO-compatible cryoprecipitate should be provided to neonates given small blood volumes and uncertain risk for passive hemolysis.[84]

Cryoprecipitate is stored frozen and must be thawed before use, it is then stored at room temperature before transfusion. Owing to its short expiration time (within 4–6 hours depending on the preparation), it should be transfused closely after being thawed. PR preparations of cryoprecipitate are now FDA-approved and offer the advantage of prolonged storage post-thaw; however, these products are expensive and understudied in neonates.[85]

Blood bank practices vary as to whether an entire unit or a small volume prepared in a syringe is dispensed for low birth weight neonates.[4] A dose of 1 to 2 units per 10 kg recipient body weight is expected to increase the fibrinogen level by 60 to 100 mg/dL and is primarily indicated in a neonate with congenital or acquired hypofibrinogenemia or dysfibrinogenemia who is bleeding or undergoing an invasive procedure. Cryoprecipitate is also a source of Factor VIII, Factor XIII, and von Willebrand Factor; however, cryoprecipitate should not be administered as factor replacement when the respective factor concentrates are available. Fibrinogen concentrates have shown promise as an alternative to cryoprecipitate in neonates undergoing cardiac surgery with cardiopulmonary bypass.[86,87]

Component Preparation of Small-Volume Aliquots

The usual dose for small-volume transfusion (10–15 mL/kg) fails to reach the usual volume of an entire unit. To address this issue and reduce blood waste, one approach is to divide RBC units into smaller, integrally attached bags (pedipacks) during manufacturing at the blood supplier.[37,88] Alternatively, an aliquot can be prepared in the blood bank by drawing off a small volume from the parent unit and transferring it into a separate container such as transfer pack or a neonatal syringe set with attached tubing.[37] When aliquots are prepared via a closed system using a sterile connection device, the parent unit retains its original expiration and the aliquot expiration is dictated by institutional policy. An aliquot may be prepared from any component type (RBC, platelets, or plasma) and must be properly labeled.

Aliquoting is a cost-effective approach that offers myriad advantages including a decreased risk TACO and a lower number of donor exposures.[37,89] The latter is accomplished by preparing serial aliquots from a single unit dedicated to one or more neonates depending on recipient weight until the unit reaches expiration (days to weeks). Aliquots prepared in syringes may be more precise in gauging the volume of the component transfused.

Special Transfusion Scenarios

1. Fresh whole blood for congenital heart disease: ABO compatible fresh whole blood (FWB) using a standard order of two units FWB (<48 hours from donation) has been used at few centers for elective cardiac operations in children younger than 2 year old. Reports of practices for over 15 years from 1995 to 2010 have shown reduced donor exposures compared with published reports of component use.[90,91] In addition, the use of FWB and pre-bypass ultrafiltration has been suggested as means for improving perioperative and postoperative outcomes. The results of a retrospective study in patients undergoing pediatric cardiac surgery requiring cardiopulmonary bypass found that FWB leads to significantly less blood exposure,

specifically in the less than 5 kg population with two-thirds of patients receiving just one exposure.[92]

2. Preparation of reconstituted whole blood for neonatal exchange transfusion: Exchange transfusion in neonates involves replacement of one or more whole blood volume(s). The most common indication for exchange transfusion in the newborn is for unconjugated hyperbilirubinemia to treat hemolytic disease of the newborn, either ABO or Rh etiology. In addition, the removal of unconjugated bilirubin, in an antibody-mediated process, exchange transfusion removes both free antibody and antibody-coated red cells. A double volume exchange removes approximately 80% to 90% of the infant's original circulating blood. The mother's serum must be screened for unexpected antibodies. RBCs selected for transfusion must be antigen negative for mother's corresponding antibodies and crossmatch compatible with maternal plasma. If maternal blood is not available, the infant's plasma (or serum) or an eluate from the infant's red cells can be used for crossmatch. For preparation of reconstituted whole blood, Group O red cells resuspended in AB plasma are commonly used. In ABO hemolytic disease, the RBCs used for exchange must be group O. If the antibody is anti-D, the red cells must be D negative. If mother and infant are ABO identical, group-specific red cells can be used. If AB plasma is not available, the choice of plasma must be ABO identical to the recipient's ABO group.

The hematocrit of the reconstituted whole blood should be 45%, if not specified by the requesting physician. The following formula can be used to determine the volume of thawed fresh frozen plasma (or thawed plasma) to be added to the RBC.

$$Total\ weight\ (Unknown) = \frac{Weight\ g \times Hct\%}{Desired\ Hct(45)\%}$$

3. ECMO: Transfusion support for ECMO in neonatal patients is covered in detail in another Chapter in this Issue.

4. ABO-incompatible heart transplant: Pediatric ABO-incompatible heart transplants (ABOiHTs) are now performed with similar outcomes to ABO-compatible transplants in an effort to increase organ availability. Owing to the newborn recipients' immunologic immaturity, lack of IHs, and serum anti-A and anti-B antibody titers usually remain low until 12 to 14 months of age, a complement system not being fully developed, therefore, the mediators of hyperacute rejection are absent during early infancy, and ABOiHTs have been performed crossing the blood group compatibility barrier.[93] There are no standard guidelines for blood product support or ABO IH titer cutoffs for transplant eligibility for these patients. A survey of transfusion support of children with ABOiHT showed widely variability and lack of standardization in practices including the choice of blood products, modifications used, titer thresholds for organ selection and medical decision points, and antibody reduction strategies among blood banks in the United States and Canada.[94]

SUMMARY

Blood bank testing and component selection practices are unique for neonates (<4 months) as compared with every other patient group. For serologic testing, ABO/Rh typing may omit the reverse testing as anti-A and anti-B antibodies in neonatal serum/plasma are of likely maternal origin. The blood bank workflows for detection of unexpected antibodies and pre-transfusion compatibility testing may differ between birth hospitals and freestanding children's hospitals, where a maternal specimen is likely to be more or less available, respectively. An evolving area of transfusion practice is the provision of group O RBC only versus group-specific RBC to neonates with the latter strategy being given increasing consideration, especially at freestanding children's hospitals. The specialized subsets of neonatal patients, such as those undergoing cardiac surgery (including ABO ABOiHTs) or receiving extracorporeal membrane oxygenation (ECMO) or exchange transfusion, require special consideration due to their exposure to high-volume transfusions. Although there is growing high-quality evidence to guide transfusion practices in neonates, it is crucial to acknowledge the unique needs of these patient groups and looking to the future to perform more clinical trials to drive evidence-based practices.

Best Practices Box

What is the current practice for neonatal blood banking?

Neonates (<4 months) have unique blood bank testing and component selection practices compared with every other patient group. Owing to the likely maternal origin of antibodies in neonatal serum/plasma, blood bank serologic testing may omit reverse typing and repeat compatibility testing on a neonatal specimen under certain circumstances. The selection and modification of blood components aims to optimize transfusion efficacy, minimize donor exposures, and mitigate potential adverse effects in the vulnerable neonatal transfusion recipient. Although there is accumulating evidence to guide blood component selection/ modification and transfusion practices in neonates, it is important to recognize the unique needs of specific neonatal patient subsets.

What changes in current practice are likely to improve outcomes?

There is a growing consideration for providing group-specific RBCs rather than group O RBCs to neonates, especially in freestanding children's hospitals. Although this strategy optimizes the availability of group O RBC, additional studies are required to understand the clinical impact in neonates.

Major Recommendations

- The direct antiglobulin test (DAT) functions poorly as a screening test for clinically significant hemolysis; a positive DAT should be interpreted in the context of ancillary laboratory data and clinical findings, whereas a negative DAT does not exclude clinically significant hemolysis.

Bibliographic Source(s)

- AABB. Standards for Blood Banks and Transfusion Services (BB/TS Standards). April 1, 2022 2022;33rd edition
- Keir A, Agpalo M, Lieberman L, Callum J. How to use: the direct antiglobulin test in newborns. *Archives of disease in childhood Education and practice edition*. Aug 2015;100(4):198 to 203. https://doi.org/10.1136/archdischild-2013-305553

DISCLOSURE

C.D. Josephson, Medtronics, unrestricted grant, Westat Consultant. R. Goel: Consultant to Westat for NHLBI Led REDS-IV-P Studies, Medical Advisory Board, Rigel Pharmaceuticals.

REFERENCES

1. Reeves HM, Goodhue Meyer E. Neonatal and pediatric blood bank practice in the United States: results from the AABB pediatric transfusion medicine subsection survey. Transfusion 2021;61(8):2265–76.

2. Roseff SD. Neonatal transfusion practice: should our policies mature with our patients? Transfusion 2011;51(5):908–13.
3. AABB. Standards for Blood Banks and Transfusion Services (BB/TS Standards). April 1, 2022 2022;33rd edition.
4. Roseff SD, Wong EC. Aabb. *Pediatric transfusion: a handbook*. Bethesda, MD: AABB; 2020.
5. New HV, Stanworth SJ. British Society for Haematology Guidelines on transfusion for fetuses, neonates and older children. Br J Haematol 2016;175:784–828. Addendum August 2020. Dec 2020;191(5):725-727.
6. Bolton-Maggs PH, Wood EM, Wiersum-Osselton JC. Wrong blood in tube - potential for serious outcomes: can it be prevented? Br J Haematol 2015;168(1):3–13.
7. Milkins C, Berryman J, Cantwell C, et al. Guidelines for pre-transfusion compatibility procedures in blood transfusion laboratories. British Committee for Standards in Haematology. Transfus Med 2013;23(1):3–35.
8. Hajjaj OI, Clarke G, Lieberman L. Immunohematology testing using umbilical cord blood: review of the literature, survey of practice and guidance development. Transfusion 2022;62(4):871–86.
9. Storry JR, Condon J, Hult AK, et al. An age-dependent ABO discrepancy between mother and baby reveals a novel A(weak) allele. Transfusion 2015;55(2):422–6.
10. Fasano RM, Luban NL. Transfusion practices. *Neonatal hematology, pathogenesis, diagnosis and management of hematologic problems*. Cambridge, UK: Cambridge University Press; 2013. p. 303–27.
11. Fu C, Lu L, Wu H, et al. Placental antibody transfer efficiency and maternal levels: specific for measles, coxsackievirus A16, enterovirus 71, poliomyelitis I-III and HIV-1 antibodies. Sci Rep 2016;6:38874.
12. Shaikh S, Sloan SR. Clearance of maternal isohemagglutinins from infant circulation (CME). Transfusion 2011;51(5):938–42.
13. Girelli G, Antoncecchi S, Casadei AM, et al. Recommendations for transfusion therapy in neonatology. Blood transfusion = Trasfusione del sangue 2015;13(3):484–97.
14. Parker V, Tormey CA. The direct antiglobulin test: indications, interpretation, and pitfalls. Arch Pathol Lab Med 2017;141(2):305–10.
15. Keir A, Agpalo M, Lieberman L, et al. How to use: the direct antiglobulin test in newborns. Archives of Disease in Childhood Education and Practice Edition 2015;100(4):198–203.
16. Crowe EP, Goel R, Andrews J, et al. Survey of newborn direct antiglobulin testing practice in United States and Canadian transfusion services. Transfusion 2021;61(4):1080–92.
17. Lieberman L, Greinacher A, Murphy MF, et al. Fetal and neonatal alloimmune thrombocytopenia: recommendations for evidence-based practice, an international approach. Br J Haematol 2019;185(3):549–62.
18. Roubinian NH, Plimier C, Woo JP, et al. Effect of donor, component, and recipient characteristics on hemoglobin increments following red blood cell transfusion. Blood 2019;134(13):1003–13.
19. Chassé M, McIntyre L, English SW, et al. Effect of blood donor characteristics on transfusion outcomes: a systematic review and meta-analysis. Transfus Med Rev 2016;30(2):69–80.
20. Kanias T, Lanteri MC, Page GP, et al. Ethnicity, sex, and age are determinants of red blood cell storage and stress hemolysis: results of the REDS-III RBC-Omics study. Blood advances 2017;1(15):1132–41.

21. D'Alessandro A, Fu X, Kanias T, et al. Donor sex, age and ethnicity impact stored red blood cell antioxidant metabolism through mechanisms in part explained by glucose 6-phosphate dehydrogenase levels and activity. Haematologica 2021; 106(5):1290–302.

22. Caram-Deelder C, Kreuger AL, Evers D, et al. Association of blood transfusion from female donors with and without a history of pregnancy with mortality among male and female transfusion recipients. JAMA 2017;318(15):1471–8.

23. Heddle NM, Cook RJ, Liu Y, et al. The association between blood donor sex and age and transfusion recipient mortality: an exploratory analysis. Transfusion 2019; 59(2):482–91.

24. Chassé M, Fergusson DA, Tinmouth A, et al. Effect of donor sex on recipient mortality in transfusion. N Engl J Med 2023;388(15):1386–95.

25. Patel RM, Lukemire J, Shenvi N, et al. Association of blood donor sex and age with outcomes in very low-birth-weight infants receiving blood transfusion. JAMA Netw Open 2021;4(9):e2123942.

26. Murphy T, Chawla A, Tucker R, et al. Impact of blood donor sex on transfusion-related outcomes in preterm infants. J Pediatr 2018;201:215–20.

27. Yoshida T, Prudent M, D'Alessandro A. Red blood cell storage lesion: causes and potential clinical consequences. Blood transfusion = Trasfusione del sangue 2019;17(1):27–52.

28. Fergusson DA, Hébert P, Hogan DL, et al. Effect of fresh red blood cell transfusions on clinical outcomes in premature, very low-birth-weight infants: the ARIPI randomized trial. JAMA 2012;308(14):1443–51.

29. Patel RM, Josephson CD. Storage age of red blood cells for transfusion of premature infants. JAMA 2013;309(6):544–5.

30. Spinella PC, Tucci M, Fergusson DA, et al. Effect of fresh vs standard-issue red blood cell transfusions on multiple organ dysfunction syndrome in critically ill pediatric patients: a randomized clinical trial. JAMA 2019;322(22):2179–90.

31. Food and Drug Administration. Dating periods for Whole Blood and blood components. 21 CFR 610.53 (b). 2023.

32. Arora S, Goel R, Al-Riyami AZ, et al. International forum on small-volume transfusions in neonates and paediatric patients: responses. Vox Sang 2023;118(3): 230–51.

33. Force CT. Circular for Information for the Use of Human Blood and Blood Components. Updated December 2021. https://www.aabb.org/docs/default-source/default-document-library/resources/circular-of-information-watermark.pdf. Accessed May 12, 2023

34. Luban NL, Strauss RG, Hume HA. Commentary on the safety of red cells preserved in extended-storage media for neonatal transfusions. Transfusion 1991; 31(3):229–35.

35. Strauss RG, Burmeister LF, Johnson K, et al. AS-1 red cells for neonatal transfusions: a randomized trial assessing donor exposure and safety. Transfusion 1996; 36(10):873–8.

36. Strauss RG, Burmeister LF, Johnson K, et al. Feasibility and safety of AS-3 red blood cells for neonatal transfusions. J Pediatr 2000;136(2):215–9.

37. Reece JT, Sesok-Pizzini D. Inventory management and product selection in pediatric blood banking. Clin Lab Med 2021;41(1):69–81.

38. Kelly MS, Benjamin DK, Puopolo KM, et al. Postnatal cytomegalovirus infection and the risk for bronchopulmonary dysplasia. JAMA Pediatr 2015;169(12): e153785.

39. Zhang L, Li Z, Han X, et al. Association between congenital cytomegalovirus infection and brain injury in neonates: a meta-analysis of cohort studies. Behav Neurol 2021;2021:9603660.
40. Ziemann M, Thiele T. Transfusion-transmitted CMV infection - current knowledge and future perspectives. Transfus Med 2017;27(4):238–48.
41. Adane T, Getawa S. Cytomegalovirus seroprevalence among blood donors: a systematic review and meta-analysis. J Int Med Res 2021;49(8). https://doi.org/10.1177/03000605211034656. 3000605211034656.
42. Das A, Munian D, Maity C, et al. Prevalence of cytomegalovirus infections in blood donors and the newborn versus utility of leukocyte-reduced blood transfusion in the premature newborn: an observation from Eastern India. Journal of Clinical Neonatology 2023;12(2):65–71.
43. Lipson SM, Shepp DH, Match ME, et al. Cytomegalovirus infectivity in whole blood following leukocyte reduction by filtration. Am J Clin Pathol 2001; 116(1):52–5.
44. Heddle NM. Universal leukoreduction and acute transfusion reactions: putting the puzzle together. Transfusion 2004;44(1):1–4.
45. Jackman RP, Deng X, Bolgiano D, et al. Leukoreduction and ultraviolet treatment reduce both the magnitude and the duration of the HLA antibody response. Transfusion 2014;54(3):672–80.
46. Weisberg SP, Staley EM, Williams LA 3rd, et al. Survey on transfusion-transmitted cytomegalovirus and cytomegalovirus disease mitigation. Arch Pathol Lab Med 2017;141(12):1705–11.
47. Heddle NM, Boeckh M, Grossman B, et al. AABB Committee Report: reducing transfusion-transmitted cytomegalovirus infections. Transfusion 2016;56(6 Pt 2): 1581–7.
48. Josephson CD, Caliendo AM, Easley KA, et al. Blood transfusion and breast milk transmission of cytomegalovirus in very low-birth-weight infants: a prospective cohort study. JAMA Pediatr 2014;168(11):1054–62.
49. Delaney M, Mayock D, Knezevic A, et al. Postnatal cytomegalovirus infection: a pilot comparative effectiveness study of transfusion safety using leukoreduced-only transfusion strategy. Transfusion 2016;56(8):1945–50.
50. Strauss RG. Optimal prevention of transfusion-transmitted cytomegalovirus (TTCMV) infection by modern leukocyte reduction alone: CMV sero/antibody-negative donors needed only for leukocyte products. Transfusion 2016;56(8): 1921–4.
51. Hu X, Hu W, Sun X, et al. Transmission of cytomegalovirus via breast milk in low birth weight and premature infants: a systematic review and meta-analysis. BMC Pediatr 2021;21(1):520.
52. Kleinman S, Stassinopoulos A. Transfusion-associated graft-versus-host disease reexamined: potential for improved prevention using a universally applied intervention. Transfusion 2018;58(11):2545–63.
53. Foukaneli T, Kerr P, Bolton-Maggs PHB. Guidelines on the use of irradiated blood components. Br J Haematol 2020;191(5):704–24.
54. Pritchard AE, Shaz BH. Survey of irradiation practice for the prevention of transfusion-associated graft-versus-host disease. Arch Pathol Lab Med 2016; 140(10):1092–7.
55. Nollet KE, Ngoma AM, Ohto H. Transfusion-associated graft-versus-host disease, transfusion-associated hyperkalemia, and potassium filtration: advancing safety and sufficiency of the blood supply. Transfus Apher Sci 2022;61(2):103408.

56. Serrano K, Chen D, Hansen AL, et al. The effect of timing of gamma-irradiation on hemolysis and potassium release in leukoreduced red cell concentrates stored in SAGM. Vox Sang 2014;106(4):379–81.
57. Saito-Benz M, Bennington K, Gray CL, et al. Effects of freshly irradiated vs irradiated and stored red blood cell transfusion on cerebral oxygenation in preterm infants: a randomized clinical trial. JAMA Pediatr 2022;176(5):e220152.
58. Cid J. Prevention of transfusion-associated graft-versus-host disease with pathogen-reduced platelets with amotosalen and ultraviolet A light: a review. Vox Sang 2017;112(7):607–13.
59. Weiskopf RB, Schnapp S, Rouine-Rapp K, et al. Extracellular potassium concentrations in red blood cell suspensions after irradiation and washing. Transfusion 2005;45(8):1295–301.
60. Burke M, Sinha P, Luban NLC, et al. Transfusion-associated hyperkalemic cardiac arrest in neonatal, infant, and pediatric patients. Frontiers in Pediatrics 2021;9:765306.
61. Honohan A, Tomson B, van der Bom J, et al. A comparison of volume-reduced versus standard HLA/HPA-matched apheresis platelets in alloimmunized adult patients. Transfusion 2012;52(4):742–51.
62. Karafin M, Fuller AK, Savage WJ, et al. The impact of apheresis platelet manipulation on corrected count increment. Transfusion 2012;52(6):1221–7.
63. Gehrie EA, Dunbar NM. Modifications to blood components: when to use them and what is the evidence? Hematol Oncol Clin N Am 2016;30(3):653–63.
64. Strauss RG. Data-driven blood banking practices for neonatal RBC transfusions. Transfusion 2000;40(12):1528–40.
65. Crawford TM, Andersen CC, Hodyl NA, et al. Effect of washed versus unwashed red blood cells on transfusion-related immune responses in preterm newborns. Clin Transl Immunology 2022;11(3):e1377.
66. Angiolillo A, Luban NL. Hemolysis following an out-of-group platelet transfusion in an 8-month-old with Langerhans cell histiocytosis. J Pediatr Hematol Oncol 2004; 26(4):267–9.
67. Weisberg SP, Shaz BH, Tumer G, et al. PAS-C platelets contain less plasma protein, lower anti-A and anti-B titers, and decreased HLA antibody specificities compared to plasma platelets. Transfusion 2018;58(4):891–5.
68. Patel RM, Josephson C. Neonatal and pediatric platelet transfusions: current concepts and controversies. Curr Opin Hematol 2019;26(6):466–72.
69. Tanaka M, Yanagisawa R, Yamanaka M, et al. Transfusion outcome for volume- and plasma-reduced platelet concentrates for pediatric patients. Transfus Apher Sci 2020;59(4):102776.
70. Schoenfeld H, Muhm M, Doepfmer UR, et al. The functional integrity of platelets in volume-reduced platelet concentrates. Anesth Analg 2005;100(1):78–81.
71. Boral LI, Staubach ZG, de Leeuw R, et al. Comparison of outcomes of group O vs non-group O premature neonates receiving group O RBC transfusions. Am J Clin Pathol 2013;140(6):780–6.
72. Thomson T, Habeeb O, Dechristopher PJ, et al. Decreased survival in necrotizing enterocolitis is significantly associated with neonatal and maternal blood group: the AB isoagglutinin hypothesis. J Perinatol : official journal of the California Perinatal Association 2012;32(8):626–30.
73. Parvizian MK, Barty R, Heddle NM, et al. Necrotizing enterocolitis and mortality after transfusion of ABO non-identical blood. Transfusion 2021;61(11):3094–103.
74. Estcourt LJ, Malouf R, Hopewell S, et al. Pathogen-reduced platelets for the prevention of bleeding. Cochrane Database Syst Rev 2017;7(7):Cd009072.

75. Lu W, Delaney M, Flegel WA, et al. How do you decide which platelet bacterial risk mitigation strategy to select for your hospital-based transfusion service? Transfusion 2020;60(4):675–81.
76. Lasky B, Nolasco J, Graff J, et al. Pathogen-reduced platelets in pediatric and neonatal patients: demographics, transfusion rates, and transfusion reactions. Transfusion 2021;61(10):2869–76.
77. Schulz WL, McPadden J, Gehrie EA, et al. Blood utilization and transfusion reactions in pediatric patients transfused with conventional or pathogen reduced platelets. J Pediatr 2019;209:220–5.
78. Amato M, Schennach H, Astl M, et al. Impact of platelet pathogen inactivation on blood component utilization and patient safety in a large Austrian Regional Medical Centre. Vox Sang 2017;112(1):47–55.
79. Nellis ME, Karam O, Valentine SL, et al. Executive summary of recommendations and expert consensus for plasma and platelet transfusion practice in critically ill children: from the transfusion and anemia EXpertise initiative-control/avoidance of bleeding (TAXI-CAB). Pediatr Crit Care Med 2022;23(1):34–51.
80. Baker JM, Shehata N, Bussel J, et al. Postnatal intervention for the treatment of FNAIT: a systematic review. J Perinatol 2019;39(10):1329–39.
81. Camazine MN, Karam O, Colvin R, et al. Outcomes related to the use of frozen plasma or pooled solvent/detergent-treated plasma in critically ill children. Pediatr Crit Care Med 2017;18(5):e215–23.
82. Spinella PC, Borasino S, Alten J. Solvent/detergent-Treated plasma in the management of pediatric patients who require replacement of multiple coagulation factors: an open-label, multicenter, post-marketing study. Frontiers in pediatrics 2020;8:572.
83. Josephson CD, Goldstein S, Askenazi D, et al. Safety and tolerability of solvent/detergent-treated plasma for pediatric patients requiring therapeutic plasma exchange: an open-label, multicenter, postmarketing study. Transfusion 2022;62(2):396–405.
84. Hadjesfandiari N, Levin E, Serrano K, et al. Risk analysis of transfusion of cryoprecipitate without consideration of ABO group. Transfusion 2021;61(1):29–34.
85. Kovacic Krizanic K, Prüller F, Rosskopf K, et al. Preparation and storage of cryoprecipitate derived from amotosalen and UVA-treated apheresis plasma and assessment of in vitro quality parameters. Pathogens 2022;11(7). https://doi.org/10.3390/pathogens11070805.
86. Downey LA, Andrews J, Hedlin H, et al. Fibrinogen concentrate as an alternative to cryoprecipitate in a postcardiopulmonary transfusion algorithm in infants undergoing cardiac surgery: a prospective randomized controlled trial. Anesth Analg 2020;130(3):740–51.
87. Tirotta CF, Lagueruela RG, Gupta A, et al. A randomized pilot trial assessing the role of human fibrinogen concentrate in decreasing cryoprecipitate use and blood loss in infants undergoing cardiopulmonary bypass. Pediatr Cardiol 2022;43(7):1444–54.
88. Gupta A, Patel R, Dyke M. Cost effective use of satellite packs in neonates: importance of birth weight. Arch Dis Child Fetal Neonatal Ed 2004;89(2):F182–3.
89. Cook S, Gunter J, Wissel M. Effective use of a strategy using assigned red cell units to limit donor exposure for neonatal patients. Transfusion 1993;33(5):379–83.
90. Jobes DR, Sesok-Pizzini D, Friedman D. Reduced transfusion requirement with use of fresh whole blood in pediatric cardiac surgical procedures. Ann Thorac Surg 2015;99(5):1706–11.

91. Sesok-Pizzini D, Friedman D, Cianfrani L, et al. How do I support a pediatric cardiac surgery program utilizing fresh whole blood? Transfusion 2019;59(4): 1180–2.
92. Valleley MS, Buckley KW, Hayes KM, et al. Are there benefits to a fresh whole blood vs. packed red blood cell cardiopulmonary bypass prime on outcomes in neonatal and pediatric cardiac surgery? J Extra Corpor Technol 2007;39(3): 168–76.
93. Foreman C, Gruenwald C, West L. ABO-incompatible heart transplantation: a perfusion strategy. Perfusion 2004;19(1):69–72.
94. Dean CL, Sullivan HC, Stowell SR, et al. Current state of transfusion practices for ABO-incompatible pediatric heart transplant patients in the United States and Canada. Transfusion 2018;58(9):2243–9.

Transfusion in Neonatal Extracorporeal Membrane Oxygenation: A Best Practice Review

Goeto Dantes, MD[a,b,*], Sarah Keene, MD[b,c,d]

KEYWORDS

• Transfusions • Neonatal • ECMO • Platelets • Blood • Coagulopathy • Thresholds

KEY POINTS

• Successful use of Extracorporeal Membrane Oxygenation (ECMO) in neonatal patients requires a thorough understanding of coagulation physiology and in-depth appreciation of transfusion medicine.
• ECMO circuitry and mechanics have dynamic impacts on blood and blood components.
• Standardized thresholds are common with an overall goal to properly support the patient while limiting excess blood product utilization; however limited evidence exists in this population and individual patient attributes often impact care.

MANUSCRIPT BODY

Since the first successful application of extracorporeal membrane oxygenation (ECMO) in a neonate in 1975, prolonged cardiorespiratory bypass support for respiratory failure in neonates has had a monumental impact on neonatal critical care.[1-4] Neonates with cardiorespiratory failure have shown improved survival through the addition of ECMO therapy as well as associated improvements in ventilatory techniques and medical management (**Table 1**).[3,5]

Encouraging as these outcomes have been, the limitations and complications of extracorporeal life support (ECLS) remain a challenge.[3,6,7] Due to the complex interaction of the blood with the mechanical elements of ECLS, a delicate balance of anticoagulation and hemostasis needs to be maintained for successful ECMO use.[7-9] This dynamic, combined with patient factors, such as intrinsic coagulopathy and the need for frequent laboratory work, has led to significant blood product use in neonates on ECMO.[10,11] Estimates of packed red blood cell (pRBC) use as high as

a Department of Surgery, Emory University, Children's Healthcare of Atlanta, Atlanta, GA, USA;
b Emory University School of Medicine, Emory University, Atlanta, GA, USA; c Department of Neonatology, Emory University, Children's Healthcare of Atlanta, Atlanta, GA, USA; d Emory + Children's Pediatric Institute, Atlanta, GA, USA
* Corresponding author. 1364 Clifton Road, Atlanta, GA 30322.
E-mail address: gdantes@emory.edu

Clin Perinatol 50 (2023) 839–852
https://doi.org/10.1016/j.clp.2023.07.003
0095-5108/23/© 2023 Elsevier Inc. All rights reserved.
perinatology.theclinics.com

	Total Runs, n	Average Run Duration, hours	Survival, N (%)
Table 1			
ECLS for neonatal respiratory failure: Diagnosis and survival			
Diagnosis			
MAS	8994	133	8418 (94)
PPHN	5077	155	3906 (77)
RDS	1555	136	1307 (84)
CDH	7786	257	3965 (51)
Sepsis	2906	144	2106 (72)

Abbreviations: CDH, Congenital Diaphragmatic Hernia; MAS, meconium aspiration syndrome; PPHN, persistent pulmonary hypertension; RDS, respiratory distress syndrome.

Data from ELSO International Summary of Statistics | ECMO | ECLS. Accessed March 31, 2023. https://www.elso.org/registry/internationalsummaryandreports/internationalsummary.aspx

40 mL/kg/day have been reported in the literature, with similar demands of platelet transfusions.[11,12] Bleeding and thrombosis are the most common causes of mortality and morbidity in neonates on ECMO with incidence as high as 60% bleeding and 44% of thrombosis.[9] A large database review of transfusion practices in US neonates demonstrated that ECMO had "the greatest incidence of transfusions and highest transfusion thresholds" within the study cohort.[13]

Historically, relatively high transfusion thresholds were established to buffer the risk of coagulopathy, bleeding, and to maintain appropriate oxygen delivery. However, recently this has been called into question.[14–16] Evidence of a lack of benefit for liberal transfusion thresholds and potential harms of the liberal use of pRBC and platelet transfusions has evolved in the neonatal literature, as echoed in adult and pediatric data. The complexity of navigating transfusion medicine for neonatal ECMO is highlighted by current heterogeneous transfusion practices among neonatal ECMO centers, relative lack of definitive data, and lack of agreement on generalizable best practice guidelines.

This article aims to provide a review the current best practice principles of transfusion medicine in neonatal ECMO by.

1. Discussing neonatal ECMO physiology that underlies the challenge of coagulopathy and bleeding during neonatal ECMO.
2. Providing a contextual understanding of historical and current pRBC, platelet, and plasma transfusion practices in neonates.
3. Reviewing the most recent literature, organizational recommendations, and best practice guidelines available for neonatal ECMO transfusion practices.
4. Discussing current clinical trials and areas where further research would be valuable.

Bleeding and clotting on extracorporeal membrane oxygenation in neonates

Mechanisms of clotting

The tension between bleeding and clotting is a primary challenge in sustaining extracorporeal life support in a neonate.[6,7] Blood exposure to the artificial surface of the extracorporeal circuit induces inflammatory and coagulative cascades, platelet adherence, endothelial dysfunction, and absorption of plasma proteins onto the circuit surfaces[17,18]. Shear stress from turbulent ECLS flow exposes collagen and von

Willebrand's factors further activating and consuming platelets. Initiation of ECMO leads to the formation of micro emboli even with systematic anticoagulation and propagation or small embolism of clots can lead to neurologic infarcts for which neonates are particularly prone.[9,19,20] In prospective work, both circuit component (40%) and patient thrombosis (7.3%) were common.[9]

Anticoagulation and associated complications

Systemic anticoagulation is necessary while on ECMO for more than just a few hours but when combined with innate fibrinolysis, consumption of thrombogenic proteins and platelet quantitative and qualitative defects leads to a significant bleeding risk.[17,21,22] Bleeding is the leading contributor to mortality in patients with ECMO.[6,8] Neonates cannulated for respiratory failure suffer from bleeding rates as high as 60%, with an up to 22% reported rate of intracranial hemorrhage.[5,8,9,20]

Packed red blood cells in neonatal extracorporeal membrane oxygenation

Physiologic principles of packed red blood cell transfusion

Many factors contribute to anemia in the neonate supported by ECLS. Sources of blood loss include frequent laboratory monitoring, ongoing cannula or surgical site bleeding, red cell deformation or hemolysis from turbulence or circuit thrombosis, as well as pathologic bleeding due to gastrointestinal, respiratory, or neurologic sources.[9,23,24] Neonates are prone to steady decreases in hemoglobin concentrations throughout their ECMO run.[14] Correcting anemia for hemodynamics as well as maintaining an adequate hemoglobin mass to support O2 delivery (DO2) for neonates being treated with ECMO is critical.[23,25,26]

Packed red blood cell transfusion thresholds

While there is general agreement that red blood cell transfusion should be provided to maintain adequate support while on ECMO, no definitive pRBC transfusion threshold has been shown to be superior.[24,27] ELSO guidelines (**Table 2**) from 2021 recommend maintaining normal to near normal hemoglobin and hematocrit while on ECMO.[28] The ELSO Red Book recommends maintaining a hematocrit >40%.[28] However, due to a growing body of evidence challenges this traditional threshold.[14,24,27,29]

First demonstrated in adults, large randomized clinical trials began to upend the practice of liberal pRBC administration in critically ill patients.[30,31] The 2007 Transfusion Strategies for patients in Pediatric Intensive Care Units (TRIPICU) a multi-center, randomized, non-inferiority trial, demonstrated no increase in adverse outcomes with maintaining hemoglobin thresholds of 7 g per deciliter (g/dL) when compared to liberal thresholds (9.5 g/dL) in critically ill children.[32] This study did not include patients on ECMO but supported applicability in the pediatric population. The 2018 Transfusion and Anemia Expertise Initiative (TAXI) guidelines upheld restrictive transfusion thresholds in pediatric patients.[33] Early trials in non ECMO neonates presented some uncertainty regarding restrictive thresholds, but recent evidence has failed to show definitive benefit in higher thresholds, consistent with adults and pediatric trials.[13,29,34–37]

PRBC transfusion requirements for the neonates on ECMO are significant, with estimates ranging as high 20 to 40 mL/kg/day of ECMO.[10–12,15,23,38] A large review of neonatal transfusion thresholds among 7 US academic and community hospitals found that neonates on ECMO support were among the highest pre-transfusion hemoglobin levels.[13] One single-center retrospective review reported pediatric (median age 2 days) patients to be exposed to a median of 267 mL/kg of pRBCs during ECMO.[26] Most of these transfusions were given for the treatment of a hematocrit of 36% and did not result in a statistically significant or clinically meaningful change in mixed venous saturation (SvO2) or cerebral near-infrared spectroscopy (NIRS).[26]

	Hemoglobin Threshold	Platelet Threshold	Plasma Transfusion
Table 2			
National consensus guidelines			
Organization	**Recommendation**	**Recommendations**	**Recommendations**
ELSO[28]	Near normal to normal hemoglobin (12–14 g/dL) & hematocrit (40%) Consider higher goal for neonates and children with cyanotic congenital heart disease or lower goal for stable, adult patients.	≥100,000 × 10⁹/L	INR: <1.5 (bleeding patient) <3 (nonbleeding patient) Fibrinogen: >150 mg/dL (bleeding patient or before surgical intervention) >100 mg/dL (nonbleeding patient)
TAXI[27,58]	In critically ill children on ECMO, there is insufficient evidence to recommend a specific RBC transfusion decision-making strategy using physiologic-based metrics and biomarkers.	≥100 × 109/L Prophylactic platelet transfusion	Data to inform decisions regarding plasma transfusions in neonates and children supported by ECMO are lacking. The decisions are complex, as anticoagulation strategies, hemostatic monitoring and plasma transfusion practices vary across institutions.

Risks associated with pRBC transfusion include volume overload, hemolytic transfusion reactions, acute lung injury, impacts of pRBC storage lesions, immunomodulation, and consequently prolonged mechanical ventilation and hospitalization.[26,39–41] Recent data suggesting risk for increased mortality from blood transfusion on ECMO is summarized in **Table 3**. Single center retrospective reviews have identified independent associations of pRBC transfusions with an increase in the number of days on ECMO and increased risk of mortality even when adjusted for the degree of illness.[12,23,25] Jackson and colleagues identified a 24% to 33% increased the risk of in-hospital mortality with each pRBC transfusion volume of 10 mL/kg/day.[25] In the only prospective pediatric study evaluating transfusion thresholds, Muszynski and colleagues again identified high transfusion requirements (roughly replacing the child entire blood volume every 3 days) and a 9% increase in odds of mortality for every 10 mL/kg/d of pRBC transfusion volume.[14]

Multiple authors have suggested that restrictive pRBC transfusion strategies may be safe in pediatric ECMO. A single center implemented of a lowered pRBC transfusion threshold showed patients had significantly lower pRBC transfusion volumes with no change in survival or complications.[15] A retrospective study of 53 pediatric and neonatal patients with ECMO, managed with restrictive protocols (threshold hemoglobin of 7 g/dL) without compromising outcomes.[42] Even lower thresholds (hematocrit between 24% and 30%) have been used in adults without the demonstration of adverse events.[16,43]

Altogether the data would suggest that existing blood transfusion thresholds may not be supported by the current data. Expert consensus from multiple organizations has recognized the need for further investigation into this topic and currently recommend (1) adoption of blood sparing and conservation procedures (2) minimizing risk of the number of donor exposures (3) using physiologic metric and biomarkers of oxygen delivery, in addition to hemoglobin concentration, to guide RBC transfusion.[27,31]

Table 3
Summary of articles on Pediatric and Neonatal pRBC Transfusion in ECMO

Article	Population	Study Type	Study Dates	Primary Outcome	Conclusion
Smith et al,[23] 2012	ECMO; Pediatric & Neonatal N = 484	Retrospective review	2001–2010	RBC transfusion volume associated mortality	Greater RBC transfusion volumes among patients supported with ECMO for non-cardiac indications are independently associated with an increase in odds of mortality.
Jackson et al,[25] 2014	ECMO; Neonates N = 825	Retrospective cohort study	1984–2011 Cohort 1 ≤ 1996 vs Cohort 2 ≥ 1997	Leukocyte-reduced blood impact on mortality and morbidity	Transfusion of non leukocyte-reduced blood is associated with an increase in mortality whereas transfusion of leukocyte-reduced blood provided no benefit
Sawyer et al,[15] 2017	ECMO; Neonates N = 72	Retrospective cohort study	2009–2014 Threshold Hct: 40% (2009–2012) vs 35% (2012–2014)	Outcomes associated with a lower reflexive red blood cell (RBC) transfusion threshold	Lower Hct threshold of 35% is associated with a reduction in RBC transfusion volume and does not appear to alter complication rates or patient outcomes
Muszynski et al,[14] 2018	ECMO; Pediatric & Neonatal N = 514	Prospective observational; subgroup analysis	2012–2016	RBC transfusion volume associated mortality	RBC transfusion volume was independently associated with odds of mortality
Keene et al,[12] 2020	ECMO; Neonatal N = 110	Retrospective review	2010–2016	RBC transfusion volume associated mortality	RBC transfusion rates are associated with in-hospital mortality among neonates receiving ECMO even with risk adjustment.

Currently a multicenter, prospective, randomized clinical Trial of Indication-based Transfusion of Red Blood Cells in ECMO (TITER) is underway (ClinicalTrials.gov identifier NCT05405426).

Platelets in neonatal extracorporeal membrane oxygenation

Platelets play a principal role in hemostasis and clot formation. Due to a combination of unique factors including limited ability to increase platelet production, neonates are more prone to developing thrombocytopenia during acute illness.[44] This becomes compounded as ECMO independently results in thrombocytopenia. Platelets have been reported to fall beginning with ECMO initiation to less than 40% of normal values.[45–47]

The clinical impact of thrombocytopenia ranges from asymptomatic to pulmonary or intracranial hemorrhage (ICH), devastating complications in the setting of ongoing anticoagulation.[44] A prospective study of neonates (non-ECMO) with severe thrombocytopenia (platelets <60 x 109/L) found an associated 82% rate of bleeding, although most was minor, and noted that the severity of thrombocytopenia did not appear to influence subsequent bleeding severity or patterns.[48] A retrospective review of 32 neonates on ECMO for persistent pulmonary hypertension associated higher rates of ICH in neonates with lower mean minimum platelet counts (37.4 x 109/L).[49] This potential morbidity as well data demonstrating an association of bleeding and subsequent mortality has led clinicians historically to be aggressive regarding platelet counts on ECMO.[9]

Platelet transfusion (**Table 4**) is currently the main treatment for thrombocytopenia in neonates and historically a near normal (>100–150 x 109/L) platelet level has been targeted during ECMO.[44,50] However, recent work in the preterm population has highlighted the lack of firm evidence that prophylactic platelet transfusion prevents bleeding, in addition to stressing the impact of platelets on thrombosis, inflammation, and other transfusion-related risks.[51,52] Ongoing development in platelet transfusion practices for critically ill neonates, on or off ECMO, has likely led to wide variability.[13,46,53–56]

Currently, ELSO and AABB (adult) guidelines recommend platelet transfusions to maintain a platelet count > 100,000 x 109/L, particularly in neonates due to the risk of ICH, with room for reduced thresholds in stable, older patients.[28,57] TAXI guidelines also recommend a transfusion threshold of >100 x 109/L (100,000/mm3).[58] This is higher than current guidelines for other critically ill neonates, with studies demonstrating ECMO infants have the greatest median pre-transfusion platelet count.[59] Using this threshold, a single site retrospective review reported neonates on ECMO for respiratory failure required a mean platelet transfusion volume of 27.4 mL/kg/day.[11]

Many platelet transfusions in neonates are administered prophylactically and as with other blood products, and higher transfusion volume are associated with increased mortality.[48,55,56] These findings are congruent with other neonatal populations, including a large, multicenter, neonatal trial that demonstrated worse outcomes (more major bleeding and death) with higher platelet transfusion thresholds (50,000 x 109/L vs 25,000 x 109/L); of note, this study did not include neonates on ECMO.[60] However, secondary analysis of the Bleeding and Thrombosis during ECMO (Bate) study, a prospective observational cohort found neonatal age groups to have increased average daily platelet transfusion volumes, and this was independently associated with increased mortality.[46] Multiple confounding variables limit definitive conclusions, given these findings are from an observational study.[61]

Duarte and colleagues presented retrospective data from pediatric and neonatal patients managed on ECMO with restrictive platelet thresholds for which most platelet

Table 4
Summary of articles on Pediatric and Neonatal Platelet Transfusion on ECMO

Article	Population	Study Type	Study Dates	Primary Outcome	Conclusion
Cashen et al,[46] 2020	ECMO; Pediatric & Neonatal Subgroup analysis N = 496	Prospective observational; subgroup analysis	2012–2014	Describe factors associated with platelet transfusion during pediatric ECMO	Platelet transfusion volume was associated with increased risk of mortality, bleeding, and thrombosis.
Keene et al,[12] 2020	ECMO; Neonatal N = 110	Retrospective review	2010–2016	Platelet transfusion volume associated mortality	Platelet transfusion rates associated with in-hospital mortality among neonates receiving ECMO.
Nellis et al,[64] 2020	ECMO; Pediatric & Neonatal Subgroup analysis of p³ T study N = 90	Prospective observational; subgroup analysis	2016–2017	Platelet Transfusion Practices amongst PICUs	ECMO patients received significantly more platelet transfusions, Median (IQR) 92 mL/kg (42–239) vs 28 mL/kg (11–68) of those not supported by ECMO ($P < .005$).
Duarte et al,[42] 2022	ECMO; Pediatric and Neonatal N = 53	Retrospective Review	2010–2019	Evaluation of restrictive (30 x 10⁹/L) transfusion thresholds	Restrictive transfusion policy, mean platelet threshold of 32 x 10⁹/L, without compromising outcome.

transfusions were administered for values below 20 x 109/L without compromising outcomes.[42] With the growing list of observational data suggesting adverse outcomes related to liberal platelet transfusion and currently no known platelet count level for which risk of bleeding is increased, more data is urgently necessary to support or revise current threshold guidelines.[62] A trial investigating ECMO hemostatic transfusions in children is being actively developed to help answer this question ECSTATIC Trial (Clinical Trial NCT05796557).

Plasma and cryoprecipitate in neonatal extracorporeal membrane oxygenation

Interaction of neonatal blood with the non-endothelial ECMO surface (eg, circuit) results in increased inflammation and activation of coagulation cascades. Fibrinogen and coagulation factors are absorbed onto mechanical surfaces which can lead to a consumptive coagulopathy.[16,17,21,48,63] Though often used for signs of bleeding or prophylactically due to laboratory indications, no prospective data has demonstrated efficacy in neonatal ECMO.

No randomized clinical trials demonstrating plasma transfusion (**Table 5**) outcomes in critically ill children are currently available, including in neonatal ECMO.[77] ELSO guidelines recommend plasma to be administered in 10 mL/kg aliquots for INR >1.5 to 2.0 or with significant bleeding and cryoprecipitate to be transfused to maintain fibrinogen levels > 100 to 150 mg/dL30. However, an international survey of anticoagulation management amongst ECMO centers demonstrates variability in indications and thresholds.[53] A prospective evaluation in 443 pediatric patients, including patients with ECLS noted that 34% of plasma transfusions were administered to patients with no bleeding or planned procedure and variability in the response to laboratory coagulopathy after plasma transfusion.[64] A single center prospective study of plasma transfusions in patients with PICU (including ECLS) noted an association with increased nosocomial infections, longer PICU length of stay and increased mortality, but with many confounders. Both plasma and cryoprecipitate have been associated with transfusion-related lung injury and adverse pulmonary reactions.[38,52]

A 2018 subgroup analysis of two pediatric prospective observational studies including 23 patients less than 1 month of age offers some insight on neonatal-specific plasma utilization in ECMO.[64] Neonates were given a median dose of 13 mL/kg plasma and comparatively received a significantly higher median dose of plasma throughout their course when compared to those not supported by ECMO. Sixty percent of transfusions were administered prophylactically and only mild reductions in INR or increases in fibrinogen were noted. This study also included a survey of ECMO centers and again noted variation in plasma transfusion practices, with 40% of centers operating without formal plasma transfusion protocols. Ultimately, comparative data regarding plasma utility in neonatal ECMO is needed.[63,64] As mentioned, experts in the field are actively engaged in trial design to help answer these important questions.

Additional considerations regarding unique blood product processing elements and discussion regarding adjuvants to coagulation factor replacement or hemostatic management play important roles for nuances in ECMO management. However, there was insufficient neonatal ECMO data on these considerations for a pertinent review at this time. As a whole, neonatal ECMO transfusions practice are closely linked to anticoagulation management and monitoring considerations.

SUMMARY

Safe neonatal ECMO management requires understanding of ECMO physiology as it relates to hemostatic pathways, including risk and benefits commonly transfused

Table 5
Summary of articles on Neonatal Plasma Transfusion on ECMO

Article	Population	Study Type	Study Dates	Primary Outcome	Conclusion
Nellis et al,[64] 2020	ECMO; Pediatric & Neonatal Subgroup analysis of PlasmaTV study N = 48	Prospective observational; subgroup analysis	April to September, 2014	Plasma Transfusion Practices amongst PICUs	Patients with ECMO received significantly more plasma, Median (IQR) 75 mL/kg (36–159) vs 20 mL/kg 10–43 of those not supported by ECMO ($P < .005$).

blood products, and up to date awareness of strides being made to close current knowledge gaps. Blood, Platelets and Plasma are commonly administered during neonatal ECMO. Thresholds for transfusion are important to maintain adequate tissue perfusion and balance bleeding risk and coagulopathy. Current transfusion guidelines are largely based on shared historical experiences and multi-institutional expert consensus, however with rapidly updated understandings of risk and benefits, there is room for additional comparative data to further define future thresholds.

Best Practices Box

What is the current practice for Red blood cell use in Neonatal ECMO for respiratory failure?

Care Path Objective(s)
- Maintain critical hemoglobin mass to support O2 content and delivery.
- Maintain appropriate hemodynamic support of intravascular neonatal volume.
- Responsible RBC utilization and limiting unnecessary neonatal transfusions/exposures.

Guideline(s)
- Extracorporeal Life Support Organization[28]: Near normal to normal hemoglobin (12–14 g/dL) & hematocrit (40%)
- Transfusion and Anemia Expertise Initiative Guidelines[27]: Evidence is insufficient to support a specific hemoglobin or hematocrit threshold for RBC transfusions

Best Practice
- At this time, though varied among centers, maintaining near-normal to normal hemoglobin and hematocrit levels is traditional practice for neonatal ECMO.
- Lowered thresholds in otherwise stable neonates with adequate evidence of tissue perfusion and hemodynamic stability should be considered to decrease RBC transfusions and exposures.

What is the current practice for Platelet use in Neonatal ECMO for respiratory failure?

Care Path Objective(s)
- Maintain adequate hemostatic balance to decrease the risk of minor and major neonatal bleeds on ECMO.
- Responsible platelet utilization to limit potential harm from further inflammatory stimulation, balance thrombotic risk and decrease unnecessary neonatal transfusions/ exposures.

Guideline(s)
- Extracorporeal Life Support Organization[28]: maintain a platelet count >100,000 cells/mm3, particularly in neonates.
- Transfusion and Anemia Expertise Initiative–Control/Avoidance of Bleeding Guidelines[58]: prophylactic platelet transfusion, $>100 \times 10^9$/L, in the absence of clinically significant bleeding is unlikely to benefit patients.

Best Practice
- Currently, maintaining platelet counts $>100 \times 10^9$/L for otherwise stable neonates with overt clinical signs of bleeding is traditional practice in ECMO.
- As there is growing evidence suggesting harm from liberal platelet use, careful consideration for lowered thresholds is actively being explored.

What is the current practice for Plasma use in Neonatal ECMO for respiratory failure?

Care Path Objective(s)
- Replace fibrinogen and coagulation factors lost through ECMO circuitry adhesion and inflammation activation as adjunctive means of maintaining hemostatic balance.
- Limit unnecessary neonatal transfusions/exposures and maintain appropriate fluid balance.

Guideline(s)
- Extracorporeal Life Support Organization[28]:
  FFP may be administered as needed if the INR is > 1.5 to 2.0 and/or if there is significant bleeding.
  Cryoprecipitate can be given if the fibrinogen level is < 100 to 150 mg/dL.

Best Practice
- Currently, maintaining INR is > 1.5 to 2.0 and fibrinogen level is < 100 to 150 mg/dL is standard practice for neonatal ECMO. However, consideration for clinical signs of bleeding, total fluid balance, limiting product exposure, responsible plasma utilization and overall circuit thrombotic burden is prudent to guide plasma use practice.

DISCLOSURE

The authors have nothing to disclose.

CONTRIBUTIONS/ROLES OF AUTHORS

All authors contributed to the study conception and design. Material preparation, data collection and analysis were performed by Goeto Dantes and Sarah Keene. The first draft of the article was written by Goeto Dantes, with revisions, corrections and final review completed by Sarah Keene. All authors read and approved the final article.

REFERENCES

1. Bartlett RH. Esperanza: the first neonatal ECMO patient. ASAIO J Am Soc Artif Intern Organs 2017;63(6):832–43.
2. Bartlett RH, Gazzaniga AB, Huxtable RF, et al. Extracorporeal circulation (ECMO) in neonatal respiratory failure. J Thorac Cardiovasc Surg 1977;74(6):826–33.
3. Gray BW, Haft JW, Hirsch JC, et al. Extracorporeal life support: experience with 2,000 patients. ASAIO J Am Soc Artif Intern Organs 2015;61(1):2–7.
4. UK collaborative randomised trial of neonatal extracorporeal membrane oxygenation. UK Collaborative ECMO Trail Group. Lancet Lond Engl 1996;348(9020):75–82.
5. ELSO International Summary of Statistics | ECMO | ECLS. Available at: https://www.elso.org/registry/internationalsummaryandreports/internationalsummary.aspx. Accessed March 31, 2023.
6. Murphy DA, Hockings LE, Andrews RK, et al. Extracorporeal membrane oxygenation-hemostatic complications. Transfus Med Rev 2015;29(2):90–101.
7. Andrews J, Winkler AM. Challenges with navigating the precarious hemostatic balance during extracorporeal life support: implications for coagulation and transfusion management. Transfus Med Rev 2016;30(4):223–9.
8. Dalton HJ, Garcia-Filion P, Holubkov R, et al. Association of bleeding and thrombosis with outcome in extracorporeal life support. Pediatr Crit Care 2015;16(2):167–74.
9. Dalton HJ, Reeder R, Garcia-Filion P, et al. Factors associated with bleeding and thrombosis in children receiving extracorporeal membrane oxygenation. Am J Respir Crit Care Med 2017;196(6):762–71.
10. Rosenberg EM, Chambers LA, Gunter JM, et al. A program to limit donor exposures to neonates undergoing extracorporeal membrane oxygenation. Pediatrics 1994;94(3):341–6.
11. Henríquez-Henríquez M, Kattan J, Chang M, et al. Blood component usage during extracorporeal membrane oxygenation: experience in 98 patients at a Latin-American tertiary hospital. Int J Artif Organs 2014;37(3):233–40.

12. Keene SD, Patel RM, Stansfield BK, et al. Blood product transfusion and mortality in neonatal extracorporeal membrane oxygenation. Transfusion (Paris) 2020;60(2): 262–8.
13. Patel RM, Hendrickson JE, Nellis ME, et al. Variation in neonatal transfusion practice. J Pediatr 2021;235:92–9.e4.
14. Muszynski JA, Reeder RW, Hall MW, et al. RBC transfusion practice in pediatric extracorporeal membrane oxygenation support. Crit Care Med 2018;46(6):e552–9.
15. Sawyer AA, Wise L, Ghosh S, et al. Comparison of transfusion thresholds during neonatal extracorporeal membrane oxygenation. Transfusion (Paris) 2017;57(9): 2115–20.
16. Cahill CM, Blumberg N, Schmidt AE, et al. Implementation of a standardized transfusion protocol for cardiac patients treated with venoarterial extracorporeal membrane oxygenation is associated with decreased blood component utilization and may improve clinical outcome. Anesth Analg 2018;126(4):1262–7.
17. Peek GJ, Firmin RK. The inflammatory and coagulative response to prolonged extracorporeal membrane oxygenation. ASAIO J Am Soc Artif Intern 1999; 45(4):250–63.
18. Millar JE, Fanning JP, McDonald CI, et al. The inflammatory response to extracorporeal membrane oxygenation (ECMO): a review of the pathophysiology. Crit Care Lond Engl 2016;20(1):387.
19. Hervey-Jumper SL, Annich GM, Yancon AR, et al. Neurological complications of extracorporeal membrane oxygenation in children. J Neurosurg Pediatr 2011; 7(4):338–44.
20. Mehta A, Ibsen LM. Neurologic complications and neurodevelopmental outcome with extracorporeal life support. World J Crit Care Med 2013;2(4):40–7.
21. Annich GM. Extracorporeal life support: the precarious balance of hemostasis. J Thromb Haemost JTH 2015;13(Suppl 1):S336–42.
22. Plötz FB, van Oeveren W, Bartlett RH, et al. Blood activation during neonatal extracorporeal life support. J Thorac Cardiovasc Surg 1993;105(5):823–32.
23. Smith A, Hardison D, Bridges B, et al. Red blood cell transfusion volume and mortality among patients receiving extracorporeal membrane oxygenation. Perfusion 2013;28(1):54–60.
24. Andrews J. Evidence for a more restrictive hematocrit trigger for neonates with respiratory failure requiring ECMO. Transfusion (Paris) 2017;57(9):2063–5.
25. Jackson HT, Oyetunji TA, Thomas A, et al. The impact of leukoreduced red blood cell transfusion on mortality of neonates undergoing extracorporeal membrane oxygenation. J Surg Res 2014;192(1):6–11.
26. Fiser RT, Irby K, Ward RM, et al. RBC transfusion in pediatric patients supported with extracorporeal membrane oxygenation: is there an impact on tissue oxygenation? Pediatr Crit Care 2014;15(9):806–13.
27. Bembea MM, Cheifetz IM, Fortenberry JD, et al. Recommendations on the indications for RBC transfusion for the critically ill child receiving support from extracorporeal membrane oxygenation, ventricular assist, and renal replacement therapy devices from the pediatric critical care transfusion and anemia Expertise initiative. Pediatr Crit Care 2018;19(9S Suppl 1):S157–62.
28. McMichael ABV, Ryerson LM, Ratano D, et al. 2021 ELSO adult and pediatric anticoagulation guidelines. ASAIO J Am Soc Artif Intern Organs 2022;68(3):303–10.
29. Whyte R, Kirpalani H. Low versus high haemoglobin concentration threshold for blood transfusion for preventing morbidity and mortality in very low birth weight infants. Cochrane Database Syst Rev 2011;11:CD000512.

30. Hébert PC, Wells G, Blajchman MA, et al. A multicenter, randomized, controlled clinical trial of transfusion requirements in critical care. Transfusion Requirements in Critical Care Investigators, Canadian Critical Care Trials Group. N Engl J Med 1999;340(6):409–17.
31. Carson JL, Guyatt G, Heddle NM, et al. Clinical practice guidelines from the AABB: red blood cell transfusion thresholds and storage. JAMA 2016;316(19):2025–35.
32. Lacroix J, Hébert PC, Hutchison JS, et al. Transfusion strategies for patients in pediatric intensive care units. N Engl J Med 2007;356(16):1609–19.
33. Valentine SL, Bembea MM, Muszynski JA, et al. Consensus recommendations for RBC transfusion practice in critically ill children from the pediatric critical care transfusion and anemia Expertise initiative. Pediatr Crit Care 2018;19(9):884–98.
34. Whyte RK, Kirpalani H, Asztalos EV, et al. Neurodevelopmental outcome of extremely low birth weight infants randomly assigned to restrictive or liberal hemoglobin thresholds for blood transfusion. Pediatrics 2009;123(1):207–13.
35. Patel RM, Knezevic A, Shenvi N, et al. Association of red blood cell transfusion, anemia, and necrotizing enterocolitis in very low-birth-weight infants. JAMA 2016;315(9):889–97.
36. Franz AR, Engel C, Bassler D, et al. Effects of liberal vs restrictive transfusion thresholds on survival and neurocognitive outcomes in extremely low-birth-weight infants: the ETTNO randomized clinical trial. JAMA 2020;324(6):560–70.
37. Kirpalani H, Bell EF, Hintz SR, et al. Higher or lower hemoglobin transfusion thresholds for preterm infants. N Engl J Med 2020;383(27):2639–51.
38. Minifee PK, Daeschner CW, Griffin MP, et al. Decreasing blood donor exposure in neonates on extracorporeal membrane oxygenation. J Pediatr Surg 1990;25(1):38–42.
39. Dodd RY. Emerging infections, transfusion safety, and epidemiology. N Engl J Med 2003;349(13):1205–6.
40. Kipps AK, Wypij D, Thiagarajan RR, et al. Blood transfusion is associated with prolonged duration of mechanical ventilation in infants undergoing reparative cardiac surgery. Pediatr Crit Care Med 2011;12(1):52–6.
41. Moore SB. Transfusion-related acute lung injury (TRALI): clinical presentation, treatment, and prognosis. Crit Care Med 2006;34(5 Suppl):S114–7.
42. Duarte CM, Lopes MI, Abecasis F. Transfusion policy in pediatric extracorporeal membrane oxygenation patients: less could be more. Perfusion 2022. https://doi.org/10.1177/02676591221105610. 2676591221105610.
43. Martucci G, Panarello G, Occhipinti G, et al. Anticoagulation and transfusions management in veno-venous extracorporeal membrane oxygenation for acute respiratory distress Syndrome: assessment of factors associated with transfusion requirements and mortality. J Intensive Care Med 2019;34(8):630–9.
44. Del Vecchio A. Evaluation and management of thrombocytopenic neonates in the intensive care unit. Early Hum Dev 2014;90(Suppl 2):S51–5.
45. Robinson TM, Kickler TS, Walker LK, et al. Effect of extracorporeal membrane oxygenation on platelets in newborns. Crit Care Med 1993;21(7):1029–34.
46. Cashen K, Dalton H, Reeder RW, et al. Platelet transfusion practice and related outcomes in pediatric extracorporeal membrane oxygenation. Pediatr Crit Care 2020;21(2):178–85.
47. Cheung PY, Sawicki G, Salas E, et al. The mechanisms of platelet dysfunction during extracorporeal membrane oxygenation in critically ill neonates. Crit Care Med 2000;28(7):2584–90.
48. Muthukumar P, Venkatesh V, Curley A, et al. Severe thrombocytopenia and patterns of bleeding in neonates: results from a prospective observational study

and implications for use of platelet transfusions. Transfus Med Oxf Engl 2012; 22(5):338–43.

49. Doymaz S, Zinger M, Sweberg T. Risk factors associated with intracranial hemorrhage in neonates with persistent pulmonary hypertension on ECMO. J Intensive Care 2015;3(1):6.

50. Christensen RD, Henry E, Del Vecchio A. Thrombocytosis and thrombocytopenia in the NICU: incidence, mechanisms and treatments. J Matern Fetal Neonatal Med 2012;25(Suppl 4):15–7.

51. Sut C, Tariket S, Aubron C, et al. The non-hemostatic aspects of transfused platelets. Front Med 2018;5:42.

52. Tariket S, Sut C, Hamzeh-Cognasse H, et al. Transfusion-related acute lung injury: transfusion, platelets and biological response modifiers. Expert Rev Hematol 2016;9(5):497–508.

53. Bembea MM, Annich G, Rycus P, et al. Variability in anticoagulation management of patients on extracorporeal membrane oxygenation: an international survey. Pediatr Crit Care Med 2013;14(2):e77–84.

54. Josephson CD, Su LL, Christensen RD, et al. Platelet transfusion practices among neonatologists in the United States and Canada: results of a survey. Pediatrics 2009;123(1):278–85.

55. Nellis ME, Karam O, Mauer E, et al. Platelet transfusion practices in critically ill children. Crit Care Med 2018;46(8):1309–17.

56. Saini A, West AN, Harrell C, et al. Platelet transfusions in the PICU: does disease severity matter? Pediatr Crit Care Med 2018;19(9):e472–8.

57. Kaufman RM, Djulbegovic B, Gernsheimer T, et al. Platelet transfusion: a clinical practice guideline from the AABB. Ann Intern Med 2015;162(3):205–13.

58. Nellis ME, Karam O, Valentine SL, et al. Executive summary of recommendations and expert consensus for plasma and platelet transfusion practice in critically ill children: from the transfusion and anemia EXpertise initiative-control/avoidance of bleeding (TAXI-CAB). Pediatr Crit Care Med 2022;23(1):34–51.

59. Nellis ME, Remy KE, Lacroix J, et al. Research priorities for plasma and platelet transfusion strategies in critically ill children: from the transfusion and anemia EXpertise initiative-control/avoidance of bleeding. Pediatr Crit Care Med 2022; 23(13 Supple 1 1S):e63–73.

60. Curley A, Stanworth SJ, Willoughby K, et al. Randomized trial of platelet-transfusion thresholds in neonates. N Engl J Med 2019;380(3):242–51.

61. MacLaren G, Monagle P. Platelet transfusion during extracorporeal membrane oxygenation: possible harm, ongoing uncertainty. Pediatr Crit Care Med 2020; 21(2):208–9.

62. Cholette JM, Muszynski JA, Ibla JC, et al. Plasma and platelet transfusions strategies in neonates and children undergoing cardiac surgery with cardiopulmonary bypass or neonates and children supported by extracorporeal membrane oxygenation: from the transfusion and anemia EXpertise initiative-control/avoidance of bleeding. Pediatr Crit Care Med 2022;23(13 Supple 1 1S):e25–36.

63. Karam O, Tucci M, Combescure C, et al. Plasma transfusion strategies for critically ill patients. Cochrane Database Syst Rev 2013;12:CD010654.

64. Nellis ME, Saini A, Spinella PC, et al. Pediatric plasma and platelet transfusions on extracorporeal membrane oxygenation: a subgroup analysis of two large international point-prevalence studies and the role of local guidelines. Pediatr Crit Care Med 2020;21(3):267–75.

Anemia, Iron Supplementation, and the Brain

Tate Gisslen, MD*, Raghavendra Rao, MD,
Michael K. Georgieff, MD

KEYWORDS

- Anemia • Brain • Neurodevelopment • Premature • Biomarkers • Iron deficiency
- Erythropoietin • Transfusion

KEY POINTS

- It is unclear what level of anemia affects brain development in human neonates.
- Phlebotomy-induced anemia likely causes brain iron deficiency because iron is prioritized to red cells over the brain.
- Erythropoiesis stimulating agents improve hematocrit and reduce the number of transfusions for preterm infants; evidence for their neurodevelopmental benefits is mixed.
- The neurodevelopmental risks of anemia at different hematocrit thresholds versus the risks and benefits of red cell transfusion (the standard treatment) are not well established.
- Although there are biomarkers of anemia and iron status in the heme compartment, reliable biomarkers of brain iron status and brain health are not available for clinical practice.

INTRODUCTION

The human brain develops rapidly in the late fetal and early neonatal period. The brain is not a homogenous organ with a single developmental trajectory. Instead, brain development can be conceptualized as a regional process with each brain region having a different developmental trajectory with different timing of onset and completion.[1] A brain region is particularly vulnerable to extrinsic environmental events such as anemia and iron deficiency during periods of its rapid development, which are often termed critical or sensitive periods.[2] Primary regions that support fundamental brain functions such as learning and memory and speed of processing begin their period of rapid development shortly before term. For example, the hippocampus has a rapid onset of differentiation starting at 28 weeks post-conceptional age, whereas myelination increases rapidly starting at 32 weeks gestation.[1] Risk factors that disrupt these

Division of Neonatology, Department of Pediatrics, University of Minnesota Medical School, Academic Office Building, 2450 Riverside Avenue, SAO-401, Minneapolis, MN 55454, USA
* Corresponding author.
E-mail address: tgisslen@umn.edu

Clin Perinatol 50 (2023) 853–868
https://doi.org/10.1016/j.clp.2023.07.009
0095-5108/23/© 2023 Elsevier Inc. All rights reserved.
perinatology.theclinics.com

processes not only cause acute dysfunction but also jeopardize brain regions that are later developing, for example, prefrontal cortex, because they rely on the integrity of connections from these more primary regions.[3] These late effects are only appreciated in long-term neurodevelopmental follow-up and are the true cost to society of early life disruption of brain development.[3]

ANEMIA AND THE DEVELOPING BRAIN

Early life anemia presents a significant risk to the developing brain because it compromises the delivery of oxygen and iron. The newborn brain is highly metabolic, using 60% of the body's total oxygen consumption rate, compared with 20% in the adult.[4] The total body oxygen consumption rate of the newborn is 2 to 2.5× greater than in adulthood. The high metabolic rate of the newborn and particularly the newborn brain derives from high-energy cost of anatomic growth and development. Thus, the brain is highly reliant on an adequate supply of substrates that support its high oxygen consumption rate including oxygen, iron, glucose, amino acids, copper, and iodine. In addition to the brain risk from reduced oxygen and iron delivery, anemia can induce a proinflammatory state in the brain.[5,6] Inflammation disrupts white matter development and neuroinflammation may contribute to developmental psychopathologies such as autism and schizophrenia.[7–9] Premature infants are at a higher risk of autism.[10] Whether inflammation due to either anemia or packed red blood cell (pRBC) transfusions contributes to this risk is unknown but the role of inflammation is suggested by preclinical models.[6,11]

Studies of infants with postnatal iron deficiency and iron deficiency anemia clearly demonstrate negative effects on short-term and long-term brain development and function.[12] Iron is a critical nutrient for the developing brain because it has a direct synthetic role in myelination,[13] energy metabolism for dendritogenesis,[14] monoamine neurotransmitter synthesis,[15] and regulation of synaptic plasticity genes through chromatin modification.[16] Infants born at term are rarely anemic although multiple gestational conditions such as moderate maternal iron deficiency,[17] intrauterine growth restriction,[18,19] maternal smoking,[20] and gestational glucose intolerance[21] compromise fetal iron stores and tissue levels.[22,23] Nonanemic term infants with low iron stores, defined as a serum ferritin less than 76 mcg/L in the neonatal period, have compromised brain function and neurodevelopment.[19,24–27]

Preterm infants are far more likely to be anemic during the time period between 28 and 40 weeks gestation because they are born with lower total body iron stores and are frequently phlebotomized.[28,29] Phlebotomy removes 3.46 mg of elemental iron per gram of hemoglobin (Hgb) lost. Because iron is prioritized to red cells over the brain, dietary and storage iron are largely used to support erythropoiesis at the expense of all other tissues including the brain.[30] Iron deficiency, irrespective of anemia, in the preterm neonate compromises neurodevelopment; adequate and timely iron supplementation is effective in promoting neurodevelopment.[31–37]

ANEMIA AND NEURODEVELOPMENT IN PRECLINICAL MODELS

Anemia has been induced by phlebotomy in developmentally appropriately aged mice to study its effects on regional brain metabolism and gene expression and behavior.[6,11,38,39] Daily phlebotomy of mice from postnatal day 3, which is the neurodevelopmental equivalent of a 26-week gestational human infant, to postnatal day 14, which is equivalent to just past term in the human, induces a state of anemia commensurate with the Hgb/hematocrit levels seen in preterm infants. Phlebotomy to a hematocrit of 25% reduces brain iron by 40%. In the hippocampus, it increases lactate levels

2-fold, reduces expression of synaptic plasticity genes such as brain-derived neurotrophic factor (BDNF) and increases vascular endothelial growth factor (VEGF) and Transferrin Receptor-1 expression.[38,39] The latter indicates that the brain is both hypoxic and iron deficient.

Phlebotomy-induced anemia (PIA) also alters the mouse hippocampal transcriptome in a dose and sex-dependent manner.[6] Male mouse pups show dysregulation of gene expression in synaptic plasticity and proinflammatory pathways when bled to target hematocrits of 25% or 18%. A similar number and type of genes are differentially expressed compared with nonbled controls at both hematocrit levels, suggesting a threshold response at a relative modest degree of anemia. In contrast, women have 91% fewer differentially expressed genes at the 25% hematocrit level compared with the men but 57% more at the 18% level. This anemia-dose dependent response in women was characterized by more proinflammatory and less synaptic plasticity pathway abnormalities compared with men.[6] The findings are of interest because of the dose-specific and sex-specific differences in cognitive performance and proinflammatory cytokines reported by Benavides and colleagues in preterm infants transfused for varying degrees of anemia.[40]

Neonatal anemia also alters adult cognitive and social-cognitive behavior in a sex and dose-dependent manner, with men with more severe anemia being the most affected.[11] The abnormality in social-cognitive behavior is characterized by a desire for social isolation and avoidance of novel environments, which can be interpreted as an anxiety or autism-like phenotype. The effect of red cell transfusion on these outcomes has not been assessed but would need to be in order to directly translate the findings in humans.[40,41]

NEONATAL ANEMIA AND ITS TREATMENT TO PROMOTE BRAIN DEVELOPMENT
Iron Supplementation

The detrimental effect of iron deficiency on the developing brain is well established. The literature on iron supplementation in the developmental window starting between 24 and 40 weeks postconceptional age is more limited. Studies in the last decade have identified this time period as perhaps the most important time to maintain iron sufficiency because it relates to the developing brain. Iron supplementation of pregnant women improves developmental outcomes at school age for offspring born at term.[42] Interestingly, postnatal iron supplementation of infants born to mothers who received placebo in the Christian and colleagues study did not improve their neurodevelopment,[43] emphasizing the critical nature of the last trimester time window for iron-dependent neurodevelopment. Infants born prematurely are by definition in the same developmental time window, which begs the question whether iron supplementation for preterm infants improves Hgb concentrations and neurodevelopment.

The literature confirms the concept that iron supplementation supports hematology and neurodevelopment. Earlier iron supplementation in preterm infants maintains better iron status and improves mental processing composite scores at 5 years of age.[33] Later gestational age preterm infants also have improved hematology outcomes and better Griffiths Mental Development Scales at 1 year of age if they are supplemented with 2 mg/kg body weight of iron versus placebo.[35] Similarly, breastfed preterm infants with birthweights between 2000 and 2500 g, whether due to prematurity or intrauterine growth restriction, have lower rates of iron deficiency and iron deficiency anemia at 6 months of age if supplemented with 1 to 2 mg/kg body of iron versus placebo.[36] The supplemented infants have less behavioral issues at 3 and 7 years.[36,37] Younger gestational age preterm infants also benefit neurodevelopmentally at 2 years of age by having greater cumulative iron dosing in the first 60 or 90 days of the newborn intensive care unit (NICU) stay.[34] Preclinical studies of iron repletion of iron-deficient animals support the concept that earlier repletion spares long-term neurodevelopment.[12]

Erythropoietin Stimulating Agents

Erythropoiesis stimulating agents (ESAs) such as erythropoietin and darbepoietin have been shown repeatedly to improve hematocrit and reduce the number of transfusions for preterm infants.[44,45] Evidence for the neurodevelopmental benefits of ESAs has been mixed.

Darbepoietin has an extended half-life that allows for less frequent dosing than erythropoietin. A randomized controlled trial (RCT) of darbepoietin was completed in preterm infants with a birth weight between 500 and 1250 g to evaluate whether transfusion need would be decreased, similar to erythropoietin, while requiring less frequent injections.[45] They compared weekly darbepoietin dosing from 48 hours of age to 35 weeks to 3 times weekly erythropoietin dosing or placebo. The primary findings confirmed decreased transfusions and donor exposures and increased hematocrit in the darbepoietin and erythropoietin groups compared with placebo. Importantly for brain development, there were no differences in mortality, retinopathy of prematurity, or intracranial hemorrhage among treatment groups. A follow-up analysis of these groups performed at 18 to 22 months suggested improved cognitive outcomes after darbepoietin and erythropoietin therapy.[46] Despite low patient numbers (27 darbepoietin, 29 erythropoietin, and 24 placebo), they found significantly higher cognitive scores in the darbepoietin and erythropoietin groups compared with placebo. There were also higher object permanence scores in both treatment groups compared with placebo and a trend toward improved language scores.

A larger RCT of preterm infants treated with high-dose erythropoietin was undertaken to explore its potential cognitive benefits therapy. In the Preterm Erythropoietin Neuroprotection Trial (PENUT), infants between 24 and 28 weeks were treated with erythropoietin starting within 48 hours of age through 32 weeks with the primary outcome of death or severe neurodevelopmental impairment that included severe cerebral palsy, Bayley Scales of Infant Development (BSID)-III cognitive score less than 70, or BSID-III motor score less than 70.[47] However, contrary to Ohls and colleagues,[46] no difference between groups was found in the primary outcome between treatment groups.

Why differing neurodevelopmental outcomes have been found between studies of ESAs is unclear. Brain iron deficiency could be a variable affecting outcomes. As discussed above, iron utilization is prioritized to red cells over other tissues including the brain.[30,48] A concern with erythropoietin therapy is that the resulting expansion of red cells could result in a relative brain iron deficiency.[49] Despite an iron supplementation protocol, infants in the PENUT study received varied amounts of iron. In a post hoc analysis, German and colleagues showed that cumulative iron dosing at 60 days of age in preterm infants from either randomized group was positively correlated with mental, motor, and language composite scores on the BSID-III.[34] Importantly, the effect was greater in infants that received erythropoietin, suggesting that augmented erythropoiesis in the erythropoietin group prioritized iron to the red cells over the brain and appropriate (higher) dosing of iron improved neurodevelopmental outcomes, consistent with preclinical literature.[30] Inability to give iron, however, did not result in worse outcomes for erythropoietin-treated infants but rather a lack of neurodevelopmental benefit. Importantly, there was not a decline of BSID-III scores at the highest doses of iron and therefore no appearance of iron toxicity.[34]

Preclinical studies have provided insight behind the mechanisms by which erythropoietin may improve neurodevelopmental outcomes. Erythropoietin is necessary for proper brain development; an absence of erythropoietin results in embryonic neurogenesis defects.[50] Erythropoietin also stimulates production of BDNF,[51,52] a hormone necessary for neuronal growth and development. Erythropoietin protects the brain during injury. It promotes neurogenesis and oligodendrocyte development following hypoxic injury,[53,54] whereas a lack of erythropoietin results in reduced cell proliferation following stroke injury.[50] Following hypoxic injury, erythropoietin has anti-inflammatory effects in the brain, reducing cytokine load and infiltrating leukocytes, and prevents brain atrophy.[55] Erythropoietin's anti-inflammatory properties may be particularly effective for neuroprotection in the treatment of neonatal anemia because we have shown increased inflammation in the neonatal hippocampus following phlebotomy-induced anemia.[6]

Erythropoietin improves brain metabolic dysfunction. Rescue treatment of PIA with erythropoietin restores hematocrit and thereby reduces the hypoxic burden as indicated by normalization of VEGF expression; however, transferrin receptor-1 expression remains elevated, indicating worsening iron deficiency.[32] The finding is consistent with shunting of dietary and storage iron preferentially into the red cells over the brain.[30,48] PIA suppresses phosphorylation of mammalian target of rapamycin pathway proteins in the hippocampus, a pathway important for monitoring critical brain metabolites such as oxygen and iron.[39] This pathway was partially rescued by erythropoietin treatment, likely improving hippocampal growth and development.

Red Blood Cell Transfusion

The standard treatment of anemia in premature infants is pRBC transfusion. More than 70% of preterm infants less than 1000 g are transfused at least once.[56] Some infants have their entire blood volume phlebotomized and replaced during as short as a 2-week period in the NICU.[29] Injuries associated with transfusion are well known in adult literature but more recent observational studies raised concerns about severe preterm injuries, including intraventricular hemorrhage and resulting neurodevelopmental deficits.[57] Although the studies of the effects of neonatal ID, with or without anemia, on the developing preterm brain are persuasive, the neurodevelopmental risks of anemia (at different hematocrit levels) versus transfusion to preterm infants are not well understood. Therefore, multiple RCTs of preterm infants sought to determine outcomes based on transfusion randomized to a higher (liberal) or lower (restrictive) threshold of anemia.[58–60]

The single-site trial of 100 newborns at the University of Iowa (Iowa study)[58] found more frequent major adverse neurologic effects (increased severe intraventricular hemorrhage and periventricular leukomalacia) during the neonatal period in the restrictive group compared with the liberal group, leading them to conclude that restrictive transfusion practices may be harmful. A multicenter RCT in Canada named the Premature Infants in Need of Transfusion (PINT) trial studied 451 infants with similar anemia thresholds for red cell transfusions.[59] This trial showed no differences in major morbidities although there was a trend toward better neurodevelopmental outcomes at 2 years of age in the infants randomized to a liberal transfusion threshold similar to the Iowa study, including the primary composite of death or neurodevelopmental impairment, cognitive delay, and neurosensory impairment.[61] The recent multicenter Transfusion of Prematures (TOP) RCT studied 1692 infants with similar anemia threshold randomization to PINT and the Iowa trials.[60] No differences in death or morbidities including neurodevelopment at 2 years were seen between the 2 groups, which differed in average threshold Hgb by ~ 20 g/L.

Long-term evaluation from the Iowa study provided a nuanced assessment of outcomes in a select group of 56 children followed up to 13 years. Their studies suggest differential neurodevelopmental outcomes related to transfusion are influenced by sex. An MRI at 12 years of age revealed no differences in brain volumes between liberal and restricted transfusion groups, although comparison to nonpreterm controls show significantly lower volumes in the liberal group but not restricted group.[62] Comparison between sexes showed that female patients in the liberal group had more structural abnormalities than male patients in the liberal group: lower volumes of multiple brain regions and total brain tissue. Comparison between liberal and restricted female patients showed lower intracranial volumes (ICV) in the liberal group and a negative correlation between cerebral white matter and mean hematocrit level, that is, higher hematocrit equaled less white matter in female patients.[63] In contrast, a lower pretransfusion Hgb for male patients correlated with lower ICV, the opposite finding from female patients.[41] When neurocognitive outcomes were measured at 8 to 15 years of age, the liberally transfused group had worse outcomes in intelligence and neuropsychological functioning compared with the restricted group.[64] However, there were also sex-specific differences. Higher pretransfusion Hgb correlated with opposite outcomes between male and female patients; female patients had a lower pooled BSID-III score with higher Hgb.[41] Overall, these studies suggest that female patients are more harmed by transfusions but male patients are more harmed by severe anemia.

The causative mechanisms differentiating male and female outcomes to level of anemia and transfusion are not well understood but inflammatory response may be involved. As described above, preclinical models of anemia demonstrate different inflammatory responses between male and female patients.[6] In neonates, multiple circulating proinflammatory cytokines increased following transfusions.[65] The cytokine responses seem to be sex-specific. In the Iowa study patients, monocyte chemoattractant protein-1 (MCP-1) increased in female neonates with cumulative transfusions but not in male neonates.[40] Importantly, MCP-1 levels negatively correlated with BSID-III cognitive scores.[40] The authors hypothesized that red cell transfusions may have caused damage to developing inflammation-sensitive structures, particularly myelin.

Taken at face value, these relatively large RCTs suggest that within the Hgb range tested, all in the anemic range, no discernible effect on gross neurodevelopmental measurements can be detected. Data from underpowered subanalyses of the clinical studies and strong corroborative support from preclinical models suggest that the effect of anemia and its treatment with pRBC transfusion may be far more complex, particularly regarding sex, than were assessed in the RCTs. Multiple reasons exist for negative neurodevelopmental outcomes in large RCTs (**Box 1**).[3] Several of these

---

Box 1
Common causes for null neurodevelopmental outcome studies in randomized controlled trials

- Wrong timing of intervention about brain development
- Target population must not already be sufficient
  - Corollary: Population must not have remained deficient after intervention
- Wrong (or insensitive) neurodevelopmental test battery
- Wrong timing of assessment about affected brain region
- Failure to identify subpopulations with opposite effects (eg, M versus F)

factors exist in the PINT and TOP trials, most notably the use of an insensitive neuro-developmental battery relative to the expected neurobiological impact and the fact that all infants were anemic and transfused, regardless of which randomization group. If the neurobiologic effects of anemia or transfusion are driven by threshold, rather than dose-response kinetics, no differentiation of outcomes would be expected between the groups.

Considered together, isolating causality of either anemia or pRBC transfusion on neurodevelopment is not possible from these 3 RCTs. The effect of anemia without transfusion on preterm neonate neurodevelopment is not possible to detect because all infants in the trials were transfused. Isolating the effect of pRBC transfusions is impossible to pick out as the root cause because of the ubiquitous existence of anemia in the population. Similarly, in trials of ESAs versus placebo, it is also hard to isolate the role of the ESAs when most if not all the infants in those trials were transfused.

To date, preclinical studies of the neurodevelopmental effects of anemia and pRBC transfusion are absent. Clues can be gathered from the single published study of anemia and neonatal transfusion where they assessed gut outcomes. MohanKumar and colleagues showed that anemia alone caused increased infiltration of macrophages into the gut.[66] Only after transfusion, however, was there a significant increase in gut inflammatory markers and susceptibility to severe gut injury. In this model, anemia seems to precondition gut tissue to inflammatory injury caused by the transfusion. A similar pathologic condition may occur in the brain; upregulation of inflammatory pathways occur in the hippocampus following phlebotomy-induced anemia.[6] However, neurologic factors such as the developmental stage of each brain region and the blood–brain barrier and blood product factors such as storage time and donor characteristics may change how transfusion affects brain injury and neurodevelopmental outcomes. Further preclinical studies in appropriate developmental models are much needed to address these questions.

Delayed Cord Clamping

Delayed clamping of the umbilical cord after birth is recommended for both preterm and full-term births. Although there is no universally accepted definition, clamping of cord 2 to 3 minutes after delivery of the infant or when cord pulsations cease is typically considered delayed cord clamping (DCC).[67] DCC allows transfer of an additional 25 to 35 mL/kg of placental blood to the infant.[67] DCC is associated with better hemodynamic stability and decreased need for transfusions in the neonatal period. A meta-analysis of 20 randomized trials involving more than 3500 infants found that compared with early cord clamping, DCC is associated with higher Hgb and serum ferritin at 6 to 10 weeks in preterm infants.[68] In full-term infants, DCC reduces the incidence of iron deficiency and iron deficiency anemia up to 1 year of age.[68–70] Additional studies have reported better myelin content in the brain regions associated with motor, visual, and sensory function[69] and better neurodevelopment, especially in boys, with DCC.[71] In regions where maternal iron deficiency in pregnancy is common, DCC is important for improving the iron status of infants.[72] Both DCC and cord milking are equally effective in this respect.[72,73]

BIOMARKERS AND BIOINDICATORS OF RISK TO THE BRAIN

A Hgb-based diagnosis and treatment strategy may not achieve neuroprotection in perinatal iron deficiency. Hgb has poor predictive sensitivity and specificity for diagnosing brain iron deficiency. Due to prioritization of available iron to the RBCs over all other organs, tissue iron deficiency, including in the developing brain, predates anemia.[23,74] The risk is highest in the perinatal period when iron needs of brain development compete with those of erythropoiesis.[48] Similarly, anemia is corrected before tissue iron deficiency during iron treatment,[75] leaving the developing brain iron-deficient for a longer duration. Data in older infants show that the treatment after the onset of anemia is inadequate for correcting the neurologic deficits,[76] likely due to persistent brain iron deficiency. A management strategy based on biomarkers of brain iron status and health in the preanemic period is therefore desirable. Some commonly used biomarkers are reviewed below.

Serum Ferritin

Serum ferritin reflects iron storage. Low serum ferritin indicates iron deficiency. A cord blood ferritin less than 35 μg/L predicts brain iron deficiency and impaired recognition memory at birth and lower psychomotor development at 1 year of age in full-term infants of diabetic mothers with iron deficiency.[77] Other studies have demonstrated that a cord blood ferritin of 75 μg/L or lesser correlates with slower auditory brainstem evoked responses, suggestive of reduced auditory tract myelination, in both full-term and preterm infants.[32,78,79] A higher cord blood serum ferritin is also associated with impaired mental and psychomotor development at 5 years of age in full-term infants.[24] A problem with serum ferritin is that levels could be falsely increased in inflammation. Iron supplementation is typically held when serum ferritin is greater than 350 to 400 μg/L.[47,49] Recent studies have demonstrated feasibility of measuring urinary ferritin in both full-term and preterm infants.[80,81] Urinary ferritin correlates with serum ferritin[80,81] and offers a noninvasive screening method. In a recent study, urine ferritin less than 12 ng/mL corrected for urine creatinine and specific gravity had 82% sensitivity and 100% specificity for detecting iron-limited erythropoiesis, with a positive predictive value of 100%.[81] However, the method requires a relatively large volume of urine and may not be sensitive in severe iron deficiency.[80]

Zinc Protoporphyrin to Heme Ratio

Zinc protoporphyrin to heme ratio (ZnPP/H) is an indicator of iron-limited erythropoiesis. When iron is not available, zinc is incorporated into the protoporphyrin molecule, leading to an increased ZnPP/H. Higher ZnPP/H indicates iron deficiency and has greater sensitivity than Hgb and serum ferritin for detecting iron deficiency. ZnPP/H from the immature erythrocyte fraction has greater sensitivity for detecting mild iron deficiency than whole blood ZnPP/H.[82] ZnPP/H is not affected by inflammation but is affected by pRBC transfusions and erythropoietin treatment. ZnPP/H deceases during the last trimester of pregnancy.[83] Cord blood ZnPP/H is higher in infants with perinatal iron deficiency.[83] A cord blood ZnPP/H greater than 118 μM/M predicts worse recognition memory at 2 months in infants with perinatal iron deficiency.[25] A serum ferritin lesser than 75 μg/L was not sensitive for such prediction in this study.[25] Similarly, a retrospective analysis demonstrated that BSID at 2 years correlate better with ZnPP/H values than serum ferritin values in extremely low gestational age neonates (ELGAN).[84]

Reticulocyte Hemoglobin

Reticulocyte Hgb, typically defined as reticulocyte Hgb content (CHr) or reticulocyte Hgb equivalent (RET-He), depending on the hematology analyzer used,[85] is an indicator of the hemoglobinization of reticulocytes and correlates with bone marrow iron level. Because reticulocytes are in the circulation only for 1 to 2 days, Ret-He provides a more real-time information on bone marrow iron status than Hgb, which is an average of the entire RBC population, each with a life span of 90 to 120 days. As in other age groups, a low CHr or RET-He is an indicator of iron deficiency in newborn infants.[86,87] Animal data show that a low RET-He also predates the onset of brain iron deficiency in the postnatal period,[88] and thus could be a biomarker of brain iron status. Our recent data in a nonhuman primate model show that Ret-He has comparable predictive accuracy for the early detection of iron deficiency and anemia as the conventional iron indices and is more sensitive than ZnPP/H.[89] Moreover, Ret-He is a component of the complete blood count in some hematology analyzers and does not require additional blood samples. Ret-He is affected less by inflammation than iron indices.[90] The small coefficient of variation also makes RET-He useful for monitoring temporal trends in the iron status of individual patients (eg, during iron or erythropoietin treatment). Reference Ret-He values for the first 90 days after birth are available from 22 to 42 weeks of gestation.[91] A value 25 pg corresponds to the 2.5 percentile in human newborn infants.[92] A Ret-He less than 29 pg had 85% sensitivity and 73% specificity for detecting iron deficiency at 3 to 4 months corrected age in one study.[93] A low RET-He can be seen in certain hemoglobinopathies, such as α and β thalassemias. Additionally, not all hematology analyzers can generate RET-He results.

Hepcidin

Similar to adults, newborn infants are capable of iron regulation through hepcidin.[70,80,94,95] Downregulation of hepcidin in iron deficiency promotes iron absorption in the gastrointestinal tract. Serum hepcidin levels correlate positively with serum ferritin, Ret-He and Hgb, and negatively with transferrin and soluble transferrin receptor in full-term and preterm infants.[70,94–96] Reference ranges for cord blood hepcidin from 24 to 42 weeks of gestation are available.[97] Serum hepcidin levels double during the first month after birth in full-term infants.[98] A level less than 16 ng/mL at 4 months of age indicates iron deficiency.[70] As with ferritin, it is possible to determine urine hepcidin. Urine hepcidin levels correlate with serum hepcidin in preterm infants.[96] A recent study showed that urine hepcidin/creatinine ratio correlates positively with serum ferritin and negatively with ZnPP/H in ELGAN.[94] A problem with hepcidin is that it is affected by erythropoietin treatment, pRBC transfusion, iron treatment, and inflammation.[86,94–97]

Biomarkers of Iron-dependent Brain Health

The above-mentioned biomarkers primarily index iron deficiency in the heme compartment and not brain iron deficiency and brain health. Molecular biomarkers of iron-dependent brain health in the blood will be better for ensuring neuroprotection during iron deficiency, especially if they can be identified in the preanemic period when the chances of preventing iron deficiency-induced adverse neurologic effects are better. Exosomes, which are small, cell-derived vesicles found in all the biofluids, carry the same classes of molecules as the parent cell and function as a snapshot of their cell of origin. Cord blood levels of exosomal contactin 2, a neural-specific glycoprotein important for brain development, are lower in newborn infants at risk for iron deficiency, especially in male infants.[99] Conversely, exosomal BDNF levels negatively correlate with serum ferritin in female infants, suggesting their biomarker potential for the early detection of iron deficiency-induced brain dysfunction in female infants.[99]

A series of proteomic and metabolomic experiments in a nonhuman primate model of infantile iron deficiency anemia from our laboratory have demonstrated the presence of neurologically important metabolites (dopamine, serotonin, and N-acetylaspartylglutamate) in the serum of infants with iron deficiency anemia.[100–102] Iron treatment led to additional changes in these metabolites.[100,101] Our recent study of paired serum and cerebrospinal fluid (CSF) in this animal model demonstrated concurrent changes in several neurologically important proteins and metabolites, such as phospholipid transfer protein, serpin family G member 1, transthyretin, and acute phase proteins in the heme and CSF compartments in the preanemic period,[102] suggesting their potential as biomarkers of brain health in early-life iron deficiency.

Biomarker-Based Iron Supplementation and Neurodevelopment

A biomarker-based standardized iron supplementation strategy has been used to minimize the risk of brain iron deficiency during erythropoietin therapy in ELGAN.[47,49] Such a strategy results in iron supplementation at a dose higher than the currently recommended dose[103] and potentially improves neurodevelopment by allowing greater cumulative iron supplementation during the first 60 days after birth.[34] However, a single biomarker may not be sensitive for both monitoring for iron deficiency and response to treatment. For example, although a serum ferritin-based strategy is useful for monitoring the risk of brain iron deficiency, it is not useful as an early biomarker of response to therapy because storage iron is the last compartment to get corrected during iron treatment, especially during active erythropoiesis.[49] An RBC-based biomarker (eg, Ret-He or reticulocyte ZnPP/H) is probably better for monitoring response to iron therapy.[83] An RBC-based biomarker also seems better than serum ferritin for monitoring brain health during iron deficiency.[104] However, additional data are needed before a biomarker-based monitoring and treatment strategy can be recommended for clinical practice. An ongoing randomized trial comparing the effects of standard iron dose (4 mg/kg/d from 2 weeks of age) with early, high iron dose (from 1 week of age and dose adjustments to maintain serum ferritin 70–400 ng/mL until 36 weeks postmenstrual age) on 2-year neurodevelopment in preterm infants (NCT04691843) may provide additional data.

FUTURE DIRECTIONS

The most urgent need is to generate biomarkers of brain risk when anemia is present in neonates and to clarify which individual characteristics, including patient sex, influence the risk to the brain by anemia and by therapy with either an ESA or pRBC transfusion. Another underexplored area is to define the risk to the brain from the heterogeneity of the transfused products. The negative effects of red cells used for transfusion can be driven by controllable factors such as length of storage, conditions of storage, and donor sex.

Best Practices Box

What is the current practice for the treatment of neonatal anemia?

There remains no standard practice, that is, no Hgb concentration target, for the treatment of neonatal anemia that protects neurologic outcomes. Although red blood cell transfusion is the standard therapy, iron supplementation and ESAs are used variably among neonatal intensive care units. The primary objective of all current interventions is limited to achieve a goal Hgb concentration because optimal neurodevelopment targeting has not been established.

What changes in current practice are likely to improve outcomes?

Preclinical and clinical evidence suggest that the treatment of anemia should be sex-specific. Therapy practices that account for patient sex will likely improve outcomes. Numerous studies have demonstrated the neuroprotective benefits of ESAs. Adequate iron supplementation is likely a necessary component. Therefore, the combined treatment will likely improve outcomes.

Major Recommendations

- Further investigation into Hgb transfusion threshold with sex-specific treatment as a primary outcome.
- Further investigation into ESAs with adequate iron supplementation as neuroprotectants.

Bibliographic Source(s)

- Bell EF, et al. Randomized trial of liberal versus restrictive guidelines for red blood cell transfusion in preterm infants. Pediatrics. 2005;115:1685 to 91.

- Kirpalani H, et al. The Premature Infants in Need of Transfusion (PINT) study: a randomized, controlled trial of a restrictive (low) versus liberal (high) transfusion threshold for extremely low birth weight infants. J Pediatr. 2006;149:301 to 307.

- Kirpalani H, et al. Higher or Lower Hemoglobin Transfusion Thresholds for Preterm Infants. N Engl J Med. 2020;383:2639 to 2651.

- Ohlsson A, Aher SM. Early erythropoiesis-stimulating agents in preterm or low birth weight infants. Cochrane Database Syst Rev. 2020;2:CD004863.

- McCarthy EK, Dempsey EM, Kiely ME. Iron supplementation in preterm and low-birth-weight infants: a systematic review of intervention studies. Nutr Rev. 2019;77:865 to 877.

DISCLOSURE

The authors have nothing to disclose.

REFERENCES

1. Thompson RA, Nelson CA. Developmental science and the media. Early brain development. Am Psychol 2001;56:5–15.
2. Hensch TK. Critical period regulation. Annu Rev Neurosci 2004;27:549–79.
3. Wachs TD, Georgieff M, Cusick S, et al. Issues in the timing of integrated early interventions: contributions from nutrition, neuroscience and psychological research. Ann N Y Acad Sci 2014;1308:89–106.
4. Kuzawa CW. Adipose tissue in human infancy and childhood: an evolutionary perspective. Am J Phys Anthropol 1998;27(Suppl):177–209.
5. Elahi S, Ertelt JM, Kinder JM, et al. Immunosuppressive CD71+ erythroid cells compromise neonatal host defence against infection. Nature 2013;504:158–62.
6. Singh G, Wallin DJ, Abrahante Llorens JE, et al. Dose- and sex-dependent effects of phlebotomy-induced anemia on the neonatal mouse hippocampal transcriptome. Pediatr Res 2022;92:712–20.
7. Hagberg H, Mallard C, Ferriero DM, et al. The role of inflammation in perinatal brain injury. Nat Rev Neurol 2015;11:192–208.
8. Brown AS. The environment and susceptibility to schizophrenia. Prog Neurobiol 2011;93:23–58.
9. Al-Haddad BJS, Oler E, Armistead B, et al. The fetal origins of mental illness. Am J Obstet Gynecol 2019;221:549–62.
10. Crump C, Sundquist J, Sundquist K. Preterm or early term birth and risk of autism. Pediatrics 2021;148. e2020032300.
11. Matveeva TM, Singh G, Gisslen TA, et al. Sex differences in adult social, cognitive, and affective behavioral deficits following neonatal phlebotomy-induced anemia in a mice. Brain Behav 2021;11:e01780.
12. Lozoff B, Beard J, Connor J, et al. Long-lasting neural and behavioral effects of early iron deficiency in infancy. Nutr Rev 2006;64:S34–43.
13. Ortiz E, Pasquini JM, Thompson K, et al. Effect of manipulation of iron storage, transport, or availability on myelin composition and brain iron content in three different animal models. J Neurosci Res 2004;77:681–9.

14. Bastian TW, von Hohenberg WC, Mickelson DJ, et al. Iron deficiency impairs developing hippocampal neuron gene expression, energy metabolism and dendrite complexity. Dev Neurosci 2016;38:264–76.

15. Unger EL, Hurst AR, Georgieff MK, et al. Behavior and monoamine deficits in pre- and perinatal iron deficiency are not corrected by early postnatal moderate or high iron diet in rats. J Nutrition 2012;142:2040–9.

16. Barks AK, Liu SX, Georgieff MK, et al. Early-life iron deficiency anemia programs the hippocampal epigenomic landscape. Nutrients 2021;13:3857.

17. Shao J, Lou J, Rao R, et al. Maternal serum ferritin concentration is positively associated with newborn iron stores in women with low ferritin status in late pregnancy. J Nutrition 2012;142:2004–9.

18. Chockalingam UM, Murphy E, Ophoven JC, et al. Cord transferrin and ferritin levels in newborn infants at risk for prenatal uteroplacental insufficiency and chronic hypoxia. J Pediatr 1987;111:283–6.

19. Siddappa AJ, Rao R, Long JD, et al. The assessment of newborn iron stores at birth: a review of the literature and standards for ferritin concentrations. Neonatology 2007;92:73–82.

20. Sweet DG, Savage G, Tubman TR, et al. Study of maternal influences on fetal iron status at term using cord blood transferrin receptors. Arch Dis Child Fetal Neonatal Ed 2001;84:F40–3.

21. Georgieff MK, Landon MB, Mills MM, et al. Abnormal iron distribution in infants of diabetic mothers: Spectrum and maternal antecedents. J Pediatr 1990;117:455–61.

22. Georgieff MK, Petry CE, Wobken JD, et al. Liver and brain iron deficiency in newborn infants with bilateral renal agenesis (Potter's syndrome). Pediatr Pathol 1996;16:509–19.

23. Petry CD, Eaton MA, Wobken JD, et al. Iron deficiency of liver, heart, and brain in newborn infants of diabetic mothers. J Pediatr 1992;121:109–14.

24. Tamura T, Goldenberg RL, Hou J, et al. Cord serum ferritin concentrations and mental and psychomotor development of children at five years of age. J Pediatr 2002;140:165–70.

25. Geng F, Mai X, Zhan J, et al. Impact of fetal-neonatal iron deficiency on recognition memory at 2 Months of age. J Pediatr 2015;167:1226–32.

26. McCarthy EK, Murray DM, Hourihane JOB, et al. Behavioral consequences at 5 y of neonatal iron deficiency in a low-risk maternal-infant cohort. Am J Clin Nutr 2021;113:1032–41.

27. Geng F, Mai X, Zhan J, et al. Timing of iron deficiency and recognition memory in infancy. Nutr Neurosci 2022;25:1–10.

28. Lorenz L, Peter A, Poets CF, et al. A review of cord blood concentrations of iron status parameters to define reference ranges for preterm infants. Neonatology 2013;104:194–202.

29. Widness JA. Pathophysiology of anemia during the neonatal period, including anemia of prematurity. NeoReviews 2008;9:e520.

30. Georgieff MK. Iron assessment to protect the developing brain. Am J Clin Nutr 2017;106:1588S–93S.

31. Armony-Sivan R, Eidelman AI, Lanir A, et al. Iron status and neurobehavioral development of premature infants. J Perinatol 2004;24:757–62.

32. Amin SB, Orlando M, Eddins A, et al. In utero iron status and auditory neural maturation in premature infants as evaluated by auditory brainstem response. J Pediatr 2010;156:377–81.

33. Steinmacher J, Pohlandt F, Bode H, et al. Randomized trial of early versus late enteral iron supplementation in infants with a birth weight of less than 1301

grams: neurocognitive development at 5.3 years' corrected age. Pediatrics 2007;120:538–46.

34. German KR, Vu PT, Comstock BA, et al, PENUT Consortium. Enteral iron supplementation in infants born extremely preterm and its positive correlation with neurodevelopment; post hoc analysis of the preterm erythropoietin neuroprotection trial randomized controlled trial. J Pediatr 2021;238:102–9.e8.

35. Luciano R, Romeo DM, Mancini G, et al. Neurological development and iron supplementation in healthy late-preterm neonates: a randomized double-blind controlled trial. Eur J Pediatr 2022;181:295–302.

36. Berglund SK, Westrup B, Hägglöf B, et al. Effects of iron supplementation of LBW infants on cognition and behavior at 3 years. Pediatrics 2013;131:47–55.

37. Berglund SK, Chmielewska A, Starnberg J, et al. Effects of iron supplementation of low-birth-weight infants on cognition and behavior at 7 years: a randomized controlled trial. Pediatr Res 2018;83:111–8.

38. Wallin DJ, Tkac I, Stucker S, et al. Phlebotomy-induced anemia alters hippocampal neurochemistry in neonatal mice. Pediatr Res 2015;77:765–71.

39. Wallin DJ, Zamora TG, Alexander M, et al. Neonatal mouse hippocampus: phlebotomy-induced anemia diminishes and treatment with erythropoietin partially rescues mammalian target of rapamycin signaling. Pediatr Res 2017; 82:501–8.

40. Benavides A, Bell EF, Georgieff MK, et al. Sex-specific cytokine responses and neurocognitive outcome after blood transfusions in preterm infants. Pediatr Res 2022;91:947–54.

41. Benavides A, Bell EF, Conrad AL, et al. Sex differences in the association of pre-transfusion hemoglobin levels with brain structure and function in the preterm infant. J Pediatr 2022;243:78–84.e5.

42. Christian P, Murray-Kolb LE, Khatry SK, et al. Prenatal micronutrient supplementation and intellectual and motor function in early school-aged children in Nepal. JAMA 2010;304:2716–23.

43. Murray-Kolb LE, Khatry SK, Katz J, et al. Preschool micronutrient supplementation effects on intellectual and motor function in school-aged Nepalese children. Arch Pediatr Adolesc Med 2012;166:404–10.

44. Juul SE, Vu PT, Comstock BA, et al. Preterm erythropoietin neuroprotection trial consortium. Effect of high-dose erythropoietin on blood transfusions in extremely low gestational age neonates: post hoc analysis of a randomized clinical trial. JAMA Pediatr 2020;174:933–43.

45. Ohls RK, Christensen RD, Kamath-Rayne BD, et al. A randomized, masked, placebo-controlled study of darbepoetin alfa in preterm infants. Pediatrics 2013;132:e119–27.

46. Ohls RK, Kamath-Rayne BD, Christensen RD, et al. Cognitive outcomes of preterm infants randomized to darbepoetin, erythropoietin, or placebo. Pediatrics 2014;133:1023–30.

47. Juul SE, Comstock BA, Wadhawan R, et al, PENUT Trial Consortium. A randomized trial of erythropoietin for neuroprotection in preterm infants. N Engl J Med 2020;382:233–43.

48. Zamora TG, Guiang SF, Widness JA, et al. Iron is prioritized to red blood cells over the brain in phlebotomized anemic newborn lambs. Pediatr Res 2016;79:922–8.

49. Siddappa AM, Olson RM, Spector M, et al. High prevalence of iron deficiency despite standardized high-dose iron supplementation during recombinant erythropoietin therapy in extremely low gestational age newborns. J Pediatr 2020;222:98–105 e3.

50. Tsai PT, Ohab JJ, Kertesz N, et al. A critical role of erythropoietin receptor in neurogenesis and post-stroke recovery. J Neurosci 2006;26:1269–74.
51. Viviani B, Bartesaghi S, Corsini E, et al. Erythropoietin protects primary hippocampal neurons increasing the expression of brain-derived neurotrophic factor. J Neurochem 2005;93:412–21.
52. Zhang F, Signore AP, Zhou Z, et al. Erythropoietin protects CA1 neurons against global cerebral ischemia in rat: potential signaling mechanisms. J Neurosci Res 2006;83:1241–51.
53. Gonzalez FF, Larpthaveesarp A, McQuillen P, et al. Erythropoietin increases neurogenesis and oligodendrogliosis of subventricular zone precursor cells after neonatal stroke. Stroke 2013;44:753–8.
54. Jantzie LL, Miller RH, Robinson S. Erythropoietin signaling promotes oligodendrocyte development following prenatal systemic hypoxic-ischemic brain injury. Pediatr Res 2013;74:658–67.
55. Sun Y, Calvert JW, Zhang JH. Neonatal hypoxia/ischemia is associated with decreased inflammatory mediators after erythropoietin administration. Stroke 2005;36:1672–8.
56. Keir AK, Yang J, Harrison A, et al, Canadian Neonatal Network. Temporal changes in blood product usage in preterm neonates born at less than 30 weeks' gestation in Canada. Transfusion 2015;55:1340–6.
57. Christensen RD, Del Vecchio A, Ilstrup SJ. More clearly defining the risks of erythrocyte transfusion in the NICU. J Matern Fetal Neonatal Med 2012;25:90–2.
58. Bell EF, Strauss RG, Widness JA, et al. Randomized trial of liberal versus restrictive guidelines for red blood cell transfusion in preterm infants. Pediatrics 2005;115:1685–91.
59. Kirpalani H, Whyte RK, Andersen C, et al. The Premature Infants in Need of Transfusion (PINT) study: a randomized, controlled trial of a restrictive (low) versus liberal (high) transfusion threshold for extremely low birth weight infants. J Pediatr 2006;149:301–7.
60. Kirpalani H, Bell EF, Hintz SR, et al, Eunice Kennedy Shriver NICHD Neonatal Research Network. Higher or lower hemoglobin transfusion thresholds for preterm infants. N Engl J Med 2020;383:2639–51.
61. Whyte RK, Kirpalani H, Asztalos EV, et al, PINTOS Study Group. Neurodevelopmental outcome of extremely low birth weight infants randomly assigned to restrictive or liberal hemoglobin thresholds for blood transfusion. Pediatrics 2009;123:207–13.
62. Nopoulos PC, Conrad AL, Bell EF, et al. Long-term outcome of brain structure in premature infants: effects of liberal vs restricted red blood cell transfusions. Arch Pediatr Adolesc Med 2011;165:443–50.
63. Benavides A, Conrad AL, Brumbaugh JE, et al. Long-term outcome of brain structure in female preterm infants: possible associations of liberal versus restrictive red blood cell transfusions. J Matern Fetal Neonatal Med 2021;34:3292–9.
64. McCoy TE, Conrad AL, Richman LC, et al. Neurocognitive profiles of preterm infants randomly assigned to lower or higher hematocrit thresholds for transfusion. Child Neuropsychol 2011;17:347–67.
65. Dani C, Poggi C, Gozzini E, et al. Red blood cell transfusions can induce proinflammatory cytokines in preterm infants. Transfusion 2017;57:1304–10.
66. MohanKumar K, Namachivayam K, Song T, et al. A murine neonatal model of necrotizing enterocolitis caused by anemia and red blood cell transfusions. Nat Commun 2019;10:3494.
67. Chaparro CM. Timing of umbilical cord clamping: effect on iron endowment of the newborn and later iron status. Nutr Rev 2011;69(Suppl 1):S30–6.

68. Zhao Y, Hou R, Zhu X, et al. Effects of delayed cord clamping on infants after neonatal period: a systematic review and meta-analysis. Int J Nurs Stud 2019; 92:97–108.

69. Mercer JS, Erickson-Owens DA, Deoni SCL, et al. Effects of delayed cord clamping on 4-month ferritin levels, brain myelin content, and neurodevelopment: a randomized controlled trial. J Pediatr 2018;203:266–272 e2.

70. Berglund SK, Chmielewska AM, Domellof M, et al. Hepcidin is a relevant iron status indicator in infancy: results from a randomized trial of early vs. delayed cord clamping. Pediatr Res 2021;89:1216–21.

71. Andersson O, Domellof M, Andersson D, et al. Effect of delayed vs early umbilical cord clamping on iron status and neurodevelopment at age 12 months: a randomized clinical trial. JAMA Pediatr 2014;168:547–54.

72. Bora R, Akhtar SS, Venkatasubramaniam A, et al. Effect of 40-cm segment umbilical cord milking on hemoglobin and serum ferritin at 6 months of age in full-term infants of anemic and non-anemic mothers. J Perinatol 2015;35:832–6.

73. Agarwal S, Jaiswal V, Singh D, et al. Randomised control trial showed that delayed cord clamping and milking resulted in no significant differences in iron stores and physical growth parameters at one year of age. Acta Paediatr 2016;105:e526–30.

74. Georgieff MK, Mills MM, Gordon K, et al. Reduced neonatal liver iron concentrations after uteroplacental insufficiency. J Pediatr 1995;127:308–14.

75. Geguchadze RN, Coe CL, Lubach GR, et al. CSF proteomic analysis reveals persistent iron deficiency-induced alterations in non-human primate infants. J Neurochem 2008;105:127–36.

76. Lukowski AF, Koss M, Burden MJ, et al. Iron deficiency in infancy and neurocognitive functioning at 19 years: evidence of long-term deficits in executive function and recognition memory. Nutr Neurosci 2010;13:54–70.

77. Siddappa AM, Georgieff MK, Wewerka S, et al. Iron deficiency alters auditory recognition memory in newborn infants of diabetic mothers. Pediatr Res 2004; 55:1034–41.

78. Amin SB, Orlando M, Wang H. Latent iron deficiency in utero is associated with abnormal auditory neural myelination in >/= 35 weeks gestational age infants. J Pediatr 2013;163:1267–71.

79. ElAlfy MS, El-Farrash RA, Taha HM, et al. Auditory brainstem response in full-term neonates born to mothers with iron deficiency anemia: relation to disease severity. J Matern Fetal Neonatal Med 2020;33:1881–8.

80. Bahr TM, Christensen RD, Ward DM, et al. Ferritin in serum and urine: a pilot study. Blood Cells Mol Dis 2019;76:59–62.

81. Gerday E, Brereton JB, Bahr TM, et al. Urinary ferritin; a potential noninvasive way to screen NICU patients for iron deficiency. J Perinatol 2021;41:1419–25.

82. Blohowiak SE, Chen ME, Repyak KS, et al. Reticulocyte enrichment of zinc protoporphyrin/heme discriminates impaired iron supply during early development. Pediatr Res 2008;64:63–7.

83. Juul SE, Zerzan JC, Strandjord TP, et al. Zinc protoporphyrin/heme as an indicator of iron status in NICU patients. J Pediatr 2003;142:273–8.

84. German KR, Vu PT, Neches S, et al. Comparison of two markers of iron sufficiency and neurodevelopmental outcomes. Early Hum Dev 2021;158:105395.

85. Piva E, Brugnara C, Spolaore F, et al. Clinical utility of reticulocyte parameters. Clin Lab Med 2015;35:133–63.

86. Lorenz L, Muller KF, Poets CF, et al. Short-term effects of blood transfusions on hepcidin in preterm infants. Neonatology 2015;108:205–10.

87. Bahr TM, Ward DM, Jia X, et al. Is the erythropoietin-erythroferrone-hepcidin axis intact in human neonates? Blood Cells Mol Dis 2021;88:102536.

88. Ennis KM, Dahl LV, Rao RB, et al. Reticulocyte hemoglobin content as an early predictive biomarker of brain iron deficiency. Pediatr Res 2018;84:765–9.

89. Rao RB, Lubach GR, Ennis-Czerniak KM, et al. Reticulocyte hemoglobin equivalent has comparable predictive accuracy as conventional serum iron indices for predicting iron deficiency and anemia in a nonhuman primate model of infantile iron deficiency. J Nutr 2023;153:148–57.

90. Ullrich C, Wu A, Armsby C, et al. Screening healthy infants for iron deficiency using reticulocyte hemoglobin content. JAMA 2005;294:924–30.

91. Christensen RD, Henry E, Bennett ST, et al. Reference intervals for reticulocyte parameters of infants during their first 90 days after birth. J Perinatol 2016; 36:61–6.

92. Lorenz L, Peter A, Arand J, et al. Reference ranges of reticulocyte haemoglobin content in preterm and term infants: a retrospective analysis. Neonatology 2017; 111:189–94.

93. Lorenz L, Arand J, Buchner K, et al. Reticulocyte haemoglobin content as a marker of iron deficiency. Arch Dis Child Fetal Neonatal Ed 2015;100:F198–202.

94. German KR, Comstock BA, Parikh P, et al. Do extremely low gestational age neonates regulate iron absorption via hepcidin? J Pediatr 2022;241:62–67 e1.

95. Berglund S, Lonnerdal B, Westrup B, et al. Effects of iron supplementation on serum hepcidin and serum erythropoietin in low-birth-weight infants. Am J Clin Nutr 2011;94:1553–61.

96. Muller KF, Lorenz L, Poets CF, et al. Hepcidin concentrations in serum and urine correlate with iron homeostasis in preterm infants. J Pediatr 2012;160: 949–953 e2.

97. Lorenz L, Herbst J, Engel C, et al. Gestational age-specific reference ranges of hepcidin in cord blood. Neonatology 2014;106:133–9.

98. Cross JH, Prentice AM, Cerami C. Hepcidin, serum iron, and transferrin Saturation in full-term and premature infants during the first month of life: a state-of-the-art review of existing evidence in humans. Curr Dev Nutr 2020;4:nzaa104.

99. Marell PS, Blohowiak SE, Evans MD, et al. Cord blood-derived exosomal CNTN2 and BDNF: potential molecular markers for brain health of neonates at risk for iron deficiency. Nutrients 2019;11:2478.

100. Sandri BJ, Lubach GR, Lock EF, et al. Early-life iron deficiency and its natural resolution are associated with altered serum metabolomic profiles in infant rhesus monkeys. J Nutr 2020;150:685–93.

101. Sandri BJ, Lubach GR, Lock EF, et al. Correcting iron deficiency anemia with iron dextran alters the serum metabolomic profile of the infant Rhesus Monkey. Am J Clin Nutr 2021;113:915–23.

102. Sandri BJ, Kim J, Lubach GR, et al. Multiomic profiling of iron-deficient infant monkeys reveals alterations in neurologically important biochemicals in serum and cerebrospinal fluid before the onset of anemia. Am J Physiol Regul Integr Comp Physiol 2022;322:R486–500.

103. Baker RD, Greer FR, Committee on Nutrition American Academy of P. Diagnosis and prevention of iron deficiency and iron-deficiency anemia in infants and young children (0-3 years of age). Pediatrics 2010;126:1040–50.

104. German K, Vu PT, Grelli KN, et al. Zinc protoporphyrin-to-heme ratio and ferritin as measures of iron sufficiency in the neonatal intensive care unit. J Pediatr 2018;194:47–53.

Patient Blood Management in Neonates

Michelle Chapman, MBBS, FRACP[a],
Amy Keir, MBBS, MPH, FRACP, PhD[a,b],*

KEYWORDS

- Neonatology • Patient blood management • Evidence-based practice

KEY POINTS

- Patient blood management (PBM) is well-established and defined in adult transfusion practice; however, it needs to be developed in neonatal transfusion practice.
- Neonatal PBM has a crucial role in supporting the implementation of the evidence base for transfusion practice.
- Key underlying principles in neonatal PBM are (1) anemia management, (2) perioperative blood conservation, and (3) appropriate blood use through the successful implementation of evidence-based transfusion guidelines.

BACKGROUND

Patient blood management (PBM) encompasses a complete evidence-based care package to improve patient outcomes by optimizing a patient's blood, minimizing blood loss, and the effective management and, when appropriate, the tolerance of anemia.[1] At a basic level, the best and safest blood for patients is their own circulating blood, hence the phrase "*keep the baby's blood in the baby.*"

Research has shown that implementing PBM guidelines in adult medicine improves patient outcomes while reducing health care costs and blood product usage.[1] The implementation of PBM in neonatal care is in its early stages,[1] and the principles used in adult PBM may not be directly transferrable to this vulnerable patient population. However, effectively using PBM in neonatal care has the potential to close the evidence-to-practice gap in neonatal transfusion practice.[2] A 2021 study of seven academic and community centers in the United States found wide variability in

[a] Department of Perinatal Medicine, Women's and Children's Hospital, 72 King William Road, North Adelaide, South Australia 5006, Australia; [b] Women's and Children's Hospital, North Adelaide and Clinical Associate Professor, Adelaide Medical School, University of Adelaide, South Australia, Australia
* Corresponding author. Department of Perinatal Medicine, Women's and Children's Hospital, 72 King William Road, North Adelaide, South Australia 5006, Australia.
E-mail address: amy.keir@adelaide.edu.au
Twitter: @AmyKKeir (A.K.)

Clin Perinatol 50 (2023) 869–879
https://doi.org/10.1016/j.clp.2023.07.004
0095-5108/23/Crown Copyright © 2023 Published by Elsevier Inc. All rights reserved.
perinatology.theclinics.com

pre-transfusion hemoglobin, platelet count, and international normalized ratio values for neonatal transfusions.[3] The investigators concluded that many neonatal transfusions were administered at thresholds greater than supported by the best available evidence.[3] They recommended increased efforts to support the translation of evidence and that PBM could be a beneficial way of doing this.[3]

In the first published review of neonatal PBM by Crighton and colleagues, the investigators did not identify any papers that examined specific neonatal PBM programs or their implementation.[1] They identified several review papers identifying critical aspects of pediatric PBM programs but not neonatal ones.[4] Since the publication of this foundational review, the Network for the Advancement of Patient Blood Management, Haemostasis and Thrombosis (NATA) published Patient Blood Management for Neonates and Children Undergoing Cardiac Surgery: 2019 NATA Guidelines.[5] Other groups have published further informative reviews in the area[6]; however, papers on specific neonatal PBM programs and their implementation and evaluation remain limited. In 2020, an Australian group published their experience implementing a PBM program.[7] This seems to be one of the few widely available and published reports on implementing a neonatal PBM program. There are, however, numerous reports of the implementation of individual components of neonatal PBM programs, which is a first practical step.

In this review, the authors explore why evidence-based guidelines are not enough, discuss the variations in neonatal transfusion practice and why this matters, and provide key updates in neonatal transfusion practice.

WHAT ABOUT EVIDENCE-BASED NEONATAL TRANSFUSION GUIDELINES?

Specific transfusion guidelines exist; in theory, they would be enough if they were consistently followed, updated rapidly with the latest evidence, and provided guidance on what to do in every clinical situation. Unfortunately, the evidence base in neonatal transfusion is limited,[2] though significant strides have been made recently with the publications of several key randomized controlled trials.[8–10] The reasons for the lack of compliance with clinical practice guidelines are complex.[11] However, a pragmatic approach to using evidence-based neonatal transfusion practice guidelines as part of a neonatal PBM program seems logical.

The Australian National Blood Authority published a neonatal and pediatric PBM guideline in 2016. This summarized current transfusion evidence and provided recommendations for clinical decisions; however, with the recent significant updates in neonatal transfusion research, they need to be updated.[12] Similar international guidelines exist in Canada and the United Kingdom; however, variability still exists.[13] If appropriately updated, these resources could provide a framework for developing local PBM guidelines. **Table 1** provides a summary of the various international transfusion guidelines that are currently available and that reflect the recent evidence updates.

VARIATIONS IN TRANSFUSION PRACTICE

Historical survey results from neonatal intensive care units in North America show varied transfusion practices.[14,15] However, despite recent advances in evidence-based transfusion thresholds, current data remain limited. Results from data collected in the United States between 2013 and 2016 showed that 80% of infants born less than 27 weeks gestation require a blood product transfusion. However, a significant proportion of these transfusions are given at thresholds above that supported by research.[3]

Table 1
Neonatal hemoglobin transfusion thresholds[12,13,32,33]

	UK British Society for Haematology			Australia National Blood Authority		Canada Canadian Paediatric Society	
	Respiratory Support		No Support	Respiratory Support	No Support	Respiratory Support	No Support
	Ventilated	Oxygen/NIPPV		Any		Oxygen>25%/NIPPV	
<24 h	<120	<120	<100	-	-	-	-
Week 1	<120	<100	<100	110–130	100–120	115	100
Week 2	<100	<95	<75–85	100–125	85–110	100	85
≥Week 3	<100	<85	<75–85	85–110	70–100	85	75

Abbreviation: NIPPV, noninvasive positive pressure ventilation.
Note: These guidelines do not necessarily include the most recent data from the TOP and ETTNO trials.
Adapted from Crighton GL, New HV, Liley HG, Stanworth SJ. PBM, what does this actually mean for neonates and infants? Transfus Med. 2018;28(2):117-131.

In 2020, collective surveys from 343 neonatal intensive care units across 18 European countries showed ongoing significant variation in transfusion practices.[16] Seventy percent of neonatal intensive care units transfused red blood cells at thresholds above those identified in the two recent randomized controlled trials, with above threshold transfusions increasing as respiratory support escalated.[16] Despite the evidence of potential harm with the use of a higher platelet transfusion threshold of 50×10^9, compared with 25×10^9 in the PLANET-2 trial, 57% transfused platelets greater than 25×10^9 in non-bleeding infants born less than 28 weeks gestation. There was increased nonadherence to platelet thresholds after ibuprofen use.[8] These findings are consistent with results from the United States, where the median platelet count at transfusion was greater than 45×10^9 in all gestational age groups.[3]

Although clear thresholds for fresh frozen plasma (FFP) transfusion do not exist, the recent European survey identified that FFP was transfused by 39% for coagulopathy without active bleeding and 25% for hypotension.[16] Both indications, however, are not currently supported by the best available evidence. Further variation in transfusion practices existed within neonatal units regarding routine coagulation testing in infants less than 32 weeks gestation, transfusion volumes and rate of infusion, the use of diuretics, and the need for fasting during transfusions.[16]

WHY DOES VARIATION IN TRANSFUSION PRACTICE MATTER?

Variation itself is not bad per se, but unwarranted or undesired variation is the concern.[17] Some variation in health care delivery is warranted and desirable, such as meeting differences in patients' health care needs or preferences.[17] The focus must be on the variation that is inexplicable by either patient need or in the cases of infants and young children, family, or caregiver preference and is therefore unwarranted. Unwarranted variation occurs when patients are exposed to actual harm from not receiving the care they need or potential harm from receiving the care they do not need and cannot benefit them.

Variation may result from *indication creep*[18] when treatment is beneficial within a narrow set of indications. In neonatal care, this potentially applies to therapeutic hypothermia for neonates with moderate to severe hypoxic-ischemic encephalopathy (HIE) when it is used in infants with mild HIE outside a trial setting, where there is currently little or no evidence of effectiveness.[19]

In the PLANET-2 trial, infants randomized to a higher platelet transfusion threshold of 50×10^9/L compared with 25×10^9/L had a higher rate of death or significant neurodevelopmental impairment at a corrected age of 2 years, which further supports evidence of harm caused by high prophylactic platelet transfusion thresholds in preterm infants.[20] Despite these findings, in a recent 2023 survey of neonatal transfusion practices across Europe, 47%–57% of neonatal units indicated using platelet count thresholds above 25×10^9/L for stable non-bleeding infants.[8] Given the strong and concerning evidence for platelet transfusion-mediated harm,[8,20] this variation and operation outside the evidence-based are concerning, though reflect the well-known time gap between getting evidence into practice.[21]

NEONATAL TRANSFUSION EVIDENCE-BASED PRACTICE: KEY UPDATES

Numerous papers review the evidence base of neonatal transfusion practice and are available for review.[2,6,22–25] The authors provide an overview of key developments in the transfusion literature across the last few years.

Red blood cells: The Effects of Transfusion Thresholds on Neurocognitive Outcomes of Extremely Low-Birth-Weight Infants (ETTNO)[10] and Transfusion of Prematures (TOP)[9] trials were published in 2020. Both randomized controlled trials were of similar design, comparing higher and lower hemoglobin thresholds for transfusing red blood cells in extremely low birth weight infants. Neither study found any difference in the primary outcome, neurodevelopmental impairment at 2 years corrected age or death before assessment, or the individual components of the primary outcome.[25] A systematic review[22] of six trials, including these two most recent randomized controlled trials ($n = 3483$ infants), found that restrictive transfusion did not increase the risk of all-cause mortality (RR, 0.99; 95% CI, 0.84–1.17; $I^2 = 0\%$; high-quality evidence) and did not increase a composite outcome of death or neurodevelopmental impairment (RR, 1.01, 95% CI, 0.93–1.09; $I^2 = 7\%$; high-quality evidence) or other serious adverse events.[22] The findings of these trials and subsequent meta-analysis contrast with the recent European survey of neonatal transfusion practice, where the majority (70%) of neonatal units used thresholds above the TOP/ETTNO restrictive thresholds, with 22% of units reporting thresholds below the restrictive thresholds.[16] These trials are discussed in detail in another Chapter in this issue.

Platelets: The PLANET-2 studies[8,20] found (1) a higher prophylactic platelet transfusion threshold (50×10^9/L) in the preterm infant is associated with significantly increased mortality or major bleeding compared with a lower one (25×10^9/L)[8] and (2) those infants randomized to the higher platelet transfusion threshold had a higher rate of death or significant neurodevelopmental impairment at a corrected age of 2 years.[20] The initial study was published in 2018, and the follow-up was in 2023. However, despite these results, the European survey of 2020 practice found that platelet transfusion thresholds above 25×10^9/L were used in 57% and 47% of neonatal intensive care unit (NICUs) for non-bleeding infants less than 28 weeks' gestational age (GA) or 28 to 32 weeks' GA, respectively.[16] It is possible that neonatal health care providers were awaiting the longer term follow-up data. However, the findings of the initial trial[8] and analyses indicated likely harm from the higher transfusion thresholds. The PLANET-2 trial is discussed in detail in another Chapter in this issue.

Fresh frozen plasma: A recent systematic review of FFP use in neonates[26] found that most FFP transfusions are administered prophylactically without evidence of active bleeding. The investigators noted that although FFP transfusions may restore coagulation test results, they do not alter the clinical outcome of neonates. Reactions following transfusions are probably underestimated in neonates, often undiagnosed, and are likely underreported. The investigators call for high-quality randomized controlled trials aiming to evaluate the effectiveness of FFP in neonates.[26] This is further supported by the recent European survey finding that 39% of neonatal units administered FFP in case of coagulopathy without bleeding and 25% of neonatal units transfusing FFP to treat hypotension, both indications not supported by the current literature.[16]

WHAT ARE THE POTENTIAL COMPONENTS OF NEONATAL PATIENT BLOOD MANAGEMENT?

High levels of evidence strongly support some of the potential components of neonatal PBM with an number of others logical and sensible (eg, use of neonatal collection tubes for sampling), and many are considered standard of practice. Individual centers need to understand their current practice and what areas may require focus to improve. The authors provide a structure for the implementation of neonatal PBM at a local level later in the paper that may be useful. Critical components of neonatal PBM adapted from Crighton and colleagues[1] may include the following.

Assessment and Management of Anemia and Anemia of Prematurity

Placental transfusion or delayed (deferred) cord clamping: A systematic review from 2018 found when comparing a total of 18 randomized controlled trials of delayed (≥30 seconds) versus early (<30 seconds) clamping in infants born less than 37 weeks' gestation, delayed (or deferred) cord clamping reduced hospital mortality.[27]

Iron supplementation: Long-term iron supplementation improves iron status and reduces iron deficiency and anemia in preterm and low birth weight infants. However, the optimum timing and duration of iron supplementation remains to be determined.[28] Despite its widespread use and recommendations for use in guidelines, high-quality evidence regarding the long-term effects of supplementation on longer term outcomes is lacking.[28,29]

Use of red blood cell transfusion thresholds using evidence-based international guidelines: There is clear evidence that guidelines restricting red blood cell transfusions can safely reduce the numbers of transfusions, volumes of blood and, potentially, donor exposure for each infant.[9,10,25,30]

Blood Conversation Strategies

These strategies are best viewed as *"keeping the baby's blood in the baby,"* and the suggested approaches include the use of neonatal collection tubes, early removal of sampling lines, point-of-care testing devices, and placental transfusion/delayed cord-clamping.[23]

Optimizing Coagulation and Hemostasis

Vitamin K supplementation

Not routinely ordering coagulation tests: Conducting conventional coagulation testing routinely on admission in NICU is not indicated as it leads to increased FFP administration without confirmed benefit.[26] The NATA Guidelines for PBM for Neonates and Children Undergoing Cardiac Surgery[24] recommend against the routine preoperative assessment of coagulation tests (eg, activated partial thromboplastin time [aPTT], PTT, or fibrinogen level) and platelet count in infants and children without a bleeding history before cardiac surgery.

Surgical and Anesthetic Techniques

Antifibrinolytics (lysine analogs): The NATA Guidelines for PBM for Neonates and Children Undergoing Cardiac Surgery[24] recommend prophylactic administration of lysine analogs, either tranexamic acid or epsilon aminocaproic acid, for all neonates undergoing surgery with cardiopulmonary bypass to reduce perioperative bleeding and transfusion.

Cell salvage: Recent technical advances have made cell salvage feasible in neonates and infants. The NATA Guidelines for PBM for Neonates and Children Undergoing Cardiac Surgery recommend its use in neonatal and pediatric cardiac surgery to reduce perioperative transfusion.

Patient and Family-Centered Decision-Making

Involvement of families and caregivers in decision-making where the evidence is lacking or uncertain is fundamental to patient and family-centered care. Input from former neonatal patients and families in the development of clinical practice guidelines is one example of how to this. Other examples included codesign of patient and family information about transfusion.

Multidisciplinary Clinical Engagement, Clinical Leadership, and Staff Education

Provision of clinical education through engagement of the multidisciplinary teams that work in neonatal units is necessary as part of a neonatal PBM program.

Audit, Review, and Quality Improvement

Audit tends only to make modest effects on health care; however, these changes can make a significant difference at a health care system level if improvements accumulate over time with repeated audit cycles.[2] Using of quality improvement approaches are more likely to have a sustained impact on clinical practice. Other system-based adjuncts to consider including clinical decision support for transfusion guidelines.[31] This approach is feasible in centers with electronic medical records allowing for clinical decision support, where "best practice alerts" that can be initiated to improve the use of blood components.[31]

EVIDENCE-BASE FOR PATIENT BLOOD MANAGEMENT PROGRAMS

PBM programs in adult health care have demonstrated improved patient morbidity and mortality while allowing prioritization of valuable resources and significantly reduced health care costs. Implementation, however, is a complex process that requires staged planning and interdisciplinary collaboration. Barriers include limited awareness of PBM, difficulty changing ingrained clinical practices and the complexities involved with managing diverse stakeholder groups.

Currently, there is a paucity of neonatal-specific PBM programs that have successfully been implemented into the clinical environment. As previously outlined, the National Blood Authority of Australia developed a neonatal and pediatric-specific PBM module providing a series of recommendations, practice points, and expert opinions.[12] In 2016 and with additions in 2020, the British Society for Haematology published an updated transfusion guideline with similar recommendations.[32,33] These guidelines cover an extensive scope of clinical practice, making direct translation to a neonatal clinical setting somewhat impractical. Instead, they can be useful by providing a strong framework from which specific local hospital guidelines can be developed.

Principals of all PBM programs revolve around three key pillars: optimizing red blood cell mass, minimizing blood loss, and managing anemia.[12] Although underlying pathophysiology within the neonatal period varies from that in adulthood, similar founding principles can be used in the development of evidence-based neonatal PBM tools. Key elements, as previously described, should include the assessment and management of anemia and anemia of prematurity, using blood conservation strategies, optimizing coagulation and hemostasis, and providing guidelines specific to surgical procedures.[12] Ensuring family-centered decision-making and multidisciplinary clinician engagement are also fundamental aspects.[12]

HOW COULD A NEONATAL PATIENT BLOOD MANAGEMENT PROGRAM BE USEFUL IN IMPROVING CARE?

As clinicians, we strive to provide evidence-based care. The development of PBM tools has only a minor role in achieving this goal. Organizational support and availability of resources are also crucial for the success of any implemented program. Overcoming variation in health care can be challenging and requires clinical leadership and focused staff education to ensure the successful adoption of evidenced-based care from those previously ingrained within practice. After implementation, audit and review of projected outcomes need to be measured to allow tailored feedback and restructuring of future implementation focus attempts.[17]

Individualized PBM tools will need to be developed as involvement and support from local stakeholders and clinical governance systems will be imperative to the success of implementation and adoption. Collaboration and sharing of developed tools between hospitals however can ensure that there is improved standardization of care for neonatal transfusions.

For evidence-based care to occur, evidence needs to be available, applicable, and acceptable, and able to be implemented, acted on and agreed to by the family or caregivers in the case of infants. Achieving this requires multiple strategies; organizational prioritization of the issue as necessary; resources to achieve the objective; systems to support clinician and consumer adoption of best practices; outcome measurement; and feedback for improvement.[17] Clinical decisions are a crucial driver of health care variation. Practice patterns of individual health care providers are influenced by their knowledge, skills, experiences, and differences in beliefs about the benefits or harms of specific interventions. Even when robust evidence on effectiveness is widely disseminated and well-publicized, practices that are at variance with the evidence may remain entrenched in some areas.

AN EXAMPLE OF THE IMPLEMENTATION OF A NEONATAL PATIENT BLOOD MANAGEMENT PROGRAM

There has been limited research published on the implementation of neonatal specific PBM programs. Flores and colleagues[7] implemented a clinical practice improvement program in an Australian neonatal intensive care unit. This specifically targeted consistency in transfusion consent and documentation using targeted clinician and parent education as well as focused follow-up surveys. Documentation standards were upheld to those set by the Australian National Safety and Quality Health Service Standards. Post-implementation auditing identified improved documentation and consent as compared with previous practice. The study was limited by incorporating only one improvement cycle, decreased clinician participation

(44%) and poor survey response rates (13%).[7] Despite these limitations, it exemplifies that implementing quality improvement programs can lead to improved neonatal transfusion practice. The resources used in this program, including a combination of neonatal-specific quality improvement tools, education, and parent/caregiver information aligned with Australian Patient Blood Management Guidelines,[12] are freely available at https://www.lifeblood.com.au/health-professionals/learn/resource-library/featured-resources.

EXAMPLES OF IMPLEMENTATION OF ONE ASPECT OF A NEONATAL PATIENT BLOOD MANAGEMENT PROGRAM

In 2021, Boston Children's Hospital published a quality improvement initiative to reduce non-indicated platelet transfusions within their neonatal intensive care unit.[34] This was based on the data from the PLANET-2 trial identifying the risk of harm with higher thresholds for platelet transfusions.[20] The quality improvement project first included a 2-year retrospective review within the unit to identify baseline rates of indicated versus non-indicated platelet transfusions. After evaluation and expert local consensus regarding accepted platelet thresholds, an electronic clinical pathway was created that identified thresholds for platelet transfusions to be used in specific clinical scenarios. As part of a 12-month prospective quality improvement cycle, targeted education and advertisement of this clinical pathway was implemented within the unit. Results showed that after only one improvement cycle, rates of non-indicated platelet transfusions decreased from a mean of 7.3 to 1.6 per month ($P < .001$) without any changes in the rates of major bleeding. Rates of platelet transfusions per 100 patient admissions also decreased from 12.5 to 2.9.[34] This is one example of how we can successfully implement PBM into the neonatal clinical environment. Although neonatal PBM encompasses all aspects of "keeping the baby's blood in the baby", targeting an individual component may improve successful implementation and allow a platform for further PBM programs to be developed.

FUTURE DIRECTIONS

Further reviews, at this stage, in neonatal PBM, are perhaps not needed. What is required are sharing neonatal PBM programs, their implementation and evaluation to allow for a better understanding of how PBM can be used effectively in neonatal care to improve patient outcomes. Recent advances in evidence supporting restrictive hemoglobin and platelet thresholds for transfusions in neonates have helped clarify previous uncertainty. Despite this, translation to clinical practice remains suboptimal. Reducing clinical practice variation requires targeted education, implementation of local guidelines and frequent reevaluation to ensure best practice is being upheld. Limitations in the evidence surrounding the optimal use of FFP, cryoprecipitate, and fibrinogen concentrate in the neonatal population provide another opportunity for future research. This is particularly pertinent where these blood products are used for non-evidence-based indications.

SUMMARY

Neonatal PBM programs represent a practical and structured way in improving the management of blood products in neonatology. In time, it seems likely that the implementation of neonatal PBM programs will be associated with improvements in clinical outcomes as well as in the rational use of blood products.

Best Practices Box

Best Practice: Neonatal Patient Blood Management

What changes in current practice are likely to improve outcomes? By following the principles of neonatal patient blood management (PBM), the evidence-based use of blood products is likely to improve and with, patient outcomes.

Major Recommendations

- Implementing neonatal PBM programs are likely to improve the evidence-based use of blood products in neonatology and, with that, patient outcomes. The three key principles are (1) anemia management, (2) perioperative blood conversation, and (3) appropriate blood product use through the successful implementation of evidence-based transfusion guidelines.

Bibliographic Source(s)

- Crighton, et al. Patient blood management, what does this actually mean for neonates and infants? Transfus Med 2018;28:117-31.
- Patel, et al. Variation in Neonatal Transfusion Practice. J Pediatr 2021;235:92-9 e4.
- Goel, et al. Pediatric Patient Blood Management Programs: Not Just Transfusing Little Adults. Transfus Med Rev 2016;30:235-41.

DISCLOSURE

The authors have nothing to disclose.

FUNDING

Amy Keir receives funding from the Australian National Health and Medical Research Council (NHMRC) (APP1161379). The contents of this paper are solely the responsibility of the individual authors and do not reflect the views of the NHMRC.

REFERENCES

1. Crighton GL, New HV, Liley HG, et al. Patient blood management, what does this actually mean for neonates and infants? Transfus Med 2018;28(2):117–31 (In eng).
2. Keir A, Grace E, Stanworth S. Closing the evidence to practice gap in neonatal transfusion medicine. Semin Fetal Neonatal Med 2021;26(1):101197.
3. Patel RM, Hendrickson JE, Nellis ME, et al. Variation in neonatal transfusion practice. J Pediatr 2021;235:92–9.e4.
4. Goel R, Cushing MM, Tobian AA. Pediatric patient blood management programs: not just transfusing little adults. Transfus Med Rev 2016;30(4):235–41.
5. Faraoni D, Meier J, New HV, et al. Patient blood management for neonates and children undergoing cardiac surgery: 2019 NATA guidelines. J Cardiothorac Vasc Anesth 2019;33(12):3249–63.
6. Gammon RR, Al-Mozain N, Auron M, et al. Transfusion therapy of neonatal and paediatric patients: they are not just little adults. Transfus Med 2022;32(6):448–59.
7. Flores CJ, Lakkundi A, McIntosh J, et al. Embedding best transfusion practice and blood management in neonatal intensive care. BMJ Open Quality 2020;9(1):e000694.

8. Curley A, Stanworth SJ, Willoughby K, et al. Randomized trial of platelet-transfusion thresholds in neonates. N Engl J Med 2018;380(3):242–51.
9. Kirpalani H, Bell EF, Hintz SR, et al. Higher or lower hemoglobin transfusion
   thresholds for preterm infants. N Engl J Med 2020;383(27):2639–51.
10. Franz AR, Engel C, Bassler D, et al. Effects of liberal vs restrictive transfusion
    thresholds on survival and neurocognitive outcomes in extremely low-birth-weight
    infants: the ETTNO randomized clinical trial. JAMA 2020;324(6):560–70 (In eng).
11. Cabana MD, Rand CS, Powe NR, et al. Why don't physicians follow clinical prac-
    tice guidelines? A framework for improvement. JAMA 1999;282(15):1458–65.
12. National Blood Authority (NBA). Patient blood management guidelines: module 6
    – Neonatal and paediatrics. Canberra (Australia): NBA; 2016.
13. Whyte RK, Jefferies AL. Red blood cell transfusion in newborn infants. Paediatr
    Child Health 2014;19(4):213–22.
14. Levy GJ, Strauss RG, Hume H, et al. National survey of neonatal transfusion prac-
    tices: I. red blood cell therapy. Pediatrics 1993;91(3):523–9 (In eng). Available at:
    http://www.ncbi.nlm.nih.gov/pubmed/8441554.
15. Strauss RG, Levy GJ, Sotelo-Avila C, et al. National survey of neonatal transfusion
    practices: II. Blood component therapy. Pediatrics 1993;91(3):530–6 (In eng).
    Available at: http://www.ncbi.nlm.nih.gov/pubmed/8382782.
16. Scrivens A, Reibel NJ, Heeger L, et al. Survey of transfusion practices in preterm
    infants in Europe. Arch Dis Child Fetal Neonatal Ed 2023. https://doi.org/10.1136/
    archdischild-2022-324619. fetalneonatal-2022-324619.
17. Duggan A, Koff E, Marshall V. Clinical variation: why it matters. Med J Aust 2016;
    205(S10):S3–4.
18. Djulbegovic B, Paul A. From efficacy to effectiveness in the face of uncertainty:
    indication creep and prevention creep. JAMA 2011;305(19):2005–6.
19. Kumar V, Singla M, Thayyil S. Cooling in mild encephalopathy: costs and perils of
    therapeutic creep. Semin Fetal Neonatal Med 2021;26(3):101244.
20. Moore CM, D'Amore A, Fustolo-Gunnink S, et al. Two-year outcomes following a
    randomised platelet transfusion trial in preterm infants. Arch Dis Child Fetal
    Neonatal Ed 2023. https://doi.org/10.1136/archdischild-2022-324915. fetalneo-
    natal-2022-324915.
21. Morris ZS, Wooding S, Grant J. The answer is 17 years, what is the question: un-
    derstanding time lags in translational research. J R Soc Med 2011;104(12):
    510–20.
22. Wang P, Wang X, Deng H, et al. Restrictive versus liberal transfusion thresholds in
    very low birth weight infants: a systematic review with meta-analysis. PLoS One
    2021;16(8):e0256810 (In eng).
23. Zerra PE, Josephson CD. Transfusion in neonatal patients: review of evidence-
    based guidelines. Clin Lab Med 2021;41(1):15–34 (In eng).
24. Boix H, Sánchez-Redondo MD, Cernada M, et al. Recommendations for transfu-
    sion of blood products in neonatology. An Pediatr (Engl Ed) 2022;97(1):60.e1–8.
25. Bell EF. Red cell transfusion thresholds for preterm infants: finally some answers.
    Arch Dis Child Fetal Neonatal Ed 2022;107(2):126–30.
26. Sokou R, Parastatidou S, Konstantinidi A, et al. Fresh frozen plasma transfusion in
    the neonatal population: a systematic review. Blood Rev 2022;55:100951.
27. Fogarty M, Osborn DA, Askie L, et al. Delayed vs early umbilical cord clamping
    for preterm infants: a systematic review and meta-analysis. Am J Obstet Gynecol
    2018;218(1):1–18 (In eng).

28. Mills RJ, Davies MW. Enteral iron supplementation in preterm and low birth weight infants. Cochrane Database Syst Rev 2012;3. https://doi.org/10.1002/14651858. CD005095.pub2.
29. McCarthy EK, Dempsey EM, Kiely ME. Iron supplementation in preterm and low-birth-weight infants: a systematic review of intervention studies. Nutr Rev 2019; 77(12):865–77 (In eng).
30. Baer VL, Henry E, Lambert DK, et al. Implementing a program to improve compliance with neonatal intensive care unit transfusion guidelines was accompanied by a reduction in transfusion rate: a pre-post analysis within a multihospital health care system. Transfusion 2011;51(2):264–9.
31. Goodnough LT, Hollenhorst MA. Clinical decision support and improved blood use in patient blood management. Hematology Am Soc Hematol Educ Program 2019;2019(1):577–82 (In eng).
32. New HV, Berryman J, Bolton-Maggs PH, et al. Guidelines on transfusion for fetuses, neonates and older children. Br J Haematol 2016;175(5):784–828 (In eng).
33. New HV, Stanworth SJ, Gottstein R, et al. British Society for Haematology Guidelines on transfusion for fetuses, neonates and older children (Br J Haematol. 2016;175:784-828). Addendum August 2020. Br J Haematol 2020;191(5):725–7 (In eng).
34. Davenport PE, Chan Yuen J, Briere J, et al. Implementation of a neonatal platelet transfusion guideline to reduce non-indicated transfusions using a quality improvement framework. J Perinatol 2021;41(6):1487–94.

Allogenic Cord Blood Transfusion in Preterm Infants

Luciana Teofili, MD, PhD[a],*, Patrizia Papacci, MD[b],
Carmen Giannantonio, MD, PhD[c], Maria Bianchi, MD, PhD[d],
Caterina Giovanna Valentini, MD, PhD[d], Giovanni Vento, MD[b]

KEYWORDS

- Preterm neonates • Blood product • Cord blood • Fetal hemoglobin
- Oxidative stress

KEY POINTS

- Repeated red blood cell (RBC) transfusions in preterm neonates cause the progressive displacement of fetal hemoglobin (HbF) by adult hemoglobin (HbA).
- Fetal and adult hemoglobin differ in oxygen affinity: the increased oxygen delivery by HbA may result at the cellular level in a condition of hyperoxia.
- Decreased levels of HbF have been associated with retinopathy of prematurity or bronchopulmonary dysplasia.
- Transfusing preterm neonates with RBC concentrates obtained from allogeneic umbilical blood is an efficacious strategy to increase hemoglobin concentration without depleting HbF.
- Studies are ongoing to demonstrate if this approach can limit the severity of diseases correlated to the oxidative damage.

INTRODUCTION

Neonatal transfusion encompasses a wide range of clinical settings with distinctive critical aspects requiring specific attentions and sometimes diverging approaches. Adverse events suffered by neonatal patients because of blood products may differ

[a] Transfusion Medicine Department, Fondazione Policlinico A. Gemelli IRCCS, Università Cattolica del Sacro Cuore, Largo Gemelli 8, Rome, Italy; [b] Neonatal Intensive Care Unit, Fondazione Policlinico A. Gemelli IRCCS, Università Cattolica del Sacro Cuore, Largo Gemelli 8, Rome, Italy; [c] Neonatal Intensive Care Unit, Fondazione Policlinico A. Gemelli IRCCS, Largo Gemelli 8, Rome, Italy; [d] Transfusion Medicine Department, Fondazione Policlinico A. Gemelli IRCCS, Largo Gemelli 8, Rome, Italy
* Corresponding author. Transfusion Medicine Department, Fondazione Policlinico A. Gemelli IRCCS, Largo Gemelli 8, Rome, Italy.
E-mail address: luciana.teofili@unicatt.it

Clin Perinatol 50 (2023) 881–893
https://doi.org/10.1016/j.clp.2023.07.005
0095-5108/23/© 2023 Elsevier Inc. All rights reserved.
perinatology.theclinics.com

from those usually reported in older patients. Moreover, particularly in preterm neonates, repeated transfusions seem to foster adverse clinical outcomes that apparently are not straightly dependent from blood products themselves. In this complex scenario, attention has been recently focused on the reciprocal changes exerted by red blood cell (RBC) transfusions on fetal hemoglobin (HbF) and adult hemoglobin (HbA) levels. Although in full-term neonates these changes constitute an acceleration of the physiologic switch from the HbF to the HbA synthesis, in preterm neonates, the substitution of HbF by HbA is aberrant. This aspect may be relevant particularly in extremely preterm neonates (ie, those born before 28 weeks of gestational age), who invariably suffer from a multifactorial severe anemia and need repeated RBC transfusions.

This review focuses on using RBC concentrates obtained from allogeneic cord blood (CB) units to transfuse preterm neonates, as a strategy to increase hemoglobin concentration without depleting the physiologic HbF reservoir. The evidence suggesting a plausible beneficial influence of this approach is discussed, and clinical experience gathered so far is reported. Finally, the necessary steps for implementing this transfusion practice and possible future directions are briefly revised.

BACKGROUND

The human hemoglobin molecules are closely related proteins formed by symmetric pairing of dimer polypeptide chains into a tetrameric functional structure: HbF consists of $\alpha_2\gamma_2$ tetramers, whereas the principal form of adult hemoglobin (HbA1) is formed of $\alpha_2\beta_2$ tetramers. Low amounts of a minor form of adult hemoglobin (HbA2) consisting of $\alpha_2\delta_2$ tetramers are also produced.[1] The HbF synthesis predominates during gestation, followed around the birth by a progressive downregulation of γ chains: the decline of γ chains is paralleled by the increased synthesis of β chains.[1,2] For clarity purpose, throughout the review, we will refer to both adult hemoglobin forms as HbA.

In 1972, Bard investigated HbF values in a series of preterm infants born at 27 to 32 weeks of gestation and observed that HbF levels in the first weeks of life did not differ remarkably from that of fetuses at the same development stage.[3] The slow transition toward the HbA synthesis accelerated as the preterm infant approached 38 weeks of postconceptional age: at this time, there was no statistical difference between the preterm-born group, who had spent several weeks of extra-uterine life, and the full-term newborn group.[2,3] These findings for the first time showed that the physiologic switching from fetal to HbA synthesis is closely connected to the developmental maturation stage and is not perturbed by the premature exposure to the extra-uterine environment.

The regulation of HbF synthesis is a field of active research due to the beneficial effect of increasing HbF levels as a treatment option for patients with sickle cell disease and β-thalassemia.[1,4] The primary driver of the switch is the transcriptional repressor BCL11 A, which occupies the γ globin gene promoters and inhibits their activity in adult erythroblasts.[5] The BCL11 A expression is primarily regulated at transcriptional level by the hypermethylated in cancer-2 (HIC2) protein, which competes with the transcription factor GATA1 and acts as a repressor of BCL11 A transcription.[6] The HbF to HbA switching is not complete or irreversible, and a proportion of erythroid cells able to synthesize HbF still persist in the adult life.[4,5]

The principal role of hemoglobins is the oxygen transport, a function that is finely tuned by allosteric forces intrinsic to the Hb molecule, or by extrinsic interactions with other molecules, such as 2,3-biphosphoglycerate (2,3 BPG), anions or protons (the Bohr effect). The γ chains have a lower binding capacity to 2,3 BPG than β chains, and the ensuing higher affinity for oxygen of HbF guarantees an adequate oxygen supply from the mother to the fetus until birth.[7] Various conditions such as anemia or cardiopulmonary diseases can induce the reactivation of HbF synthesis also in postnatal life.[8] In these situations, an expansion of HbF erythroid cell population is usually observed, conceivably due to the direct activation of γ-globin expression by the hypoxia-inducible factor 1α.[9] This physiologic response, known as "stress erythropoiesis," emphasizes HbF as a mediator of the adaptation to hypoxia.[8,9] As purveyor of the vasoactive mediator nitric oxide (NO), Hb is also an important regulator of the microcirculatory blood flow. Two main mechanisms have been identified for the NO release from hemoglobin. The first pathway consists of an oxidative denitrosylation reaction in which nitrite react in parallel with both oxyhemoglobin and deoxyhemoglobin at the heme iron sites.[10] Oxidants generated by the oxyhemoglobin reaction oxidizes the ferrous heme of iron-nitrosyl-hemoglobin produced by the deoxyhemoglobin reaction to NO-methemoglobin, which subsequently releases free NO.[10] In the other pathway, NO binds reversibly to the thiol group of cysteine residue in position 93 (Cys93) of β and γ chains, forming the stable SNO carrier S-nitrosohemoglobin (SNO-Hb).[11] This reaction is allosterically mediated because Cys93 reactivity significantly increases from the oxygenated to the deoxygenated Hb. Indeed, as the oxygen is released to peripheral tissues, the ensuing SNO shuttling from RBCs to the vessel wall modulates blood flow.[11] Although controversial evidence has been generated, the allosteric linkage of oxygen and SNO delivery has been proposed as the basis for the hypoxia-dependent microcirculatory blood flow regulation.[11–13] The C93 A mouse model expressing a hybrid form of mutant human Hb (consisting of a dimer of 2 human α chains coupled with a dimer composed by one β chain of mouse origin and one β chain of human origin in which β-globin Cys93 was substituted by an alanine), shows a severe impairment of microcirculatory blood flow and tissue oxygenation, higher lethality at birth, poor short-term ventilation potential, and compensatory increase of HbF levels.[11,14]

LOW FETAL HEMOGLOBIN LEVELS AND COMORBIDITIES IN PRETERM INFANTS

In 2002, De Halleux and colleagues explored HbF levels before and after transfusions in preterm neonates.[15] Eleven infants with gestational age of 23 to 27 weeks were investigated. The percentage of HbF on total Hb was 92.9 ± 1.1% before and 42.6 ± 5.7% after transfusion. Interestingly, the authors also calculated the increase of P_{50} values (ie, the oxygen tension at 50% saturation of Hb at standard temperature and pH) after transfusion and suggested lowering oxygen saturation targets in neonates on oxygen therapy receiving RBC transfusions.[15] Several subsequent studies have largely confirmed that RBC transfusions are the main cause of HbF depletion in preterm neonates.[16–19] The decline of HbF values after each RBC transfusion is predictable according to the equation: postHbF = $(0.6502 \times \text{preHbF}) - 9.841$.[19]

The association between low-HbF levels and poor outcome in preterm neonates has also been explored in retrospective and prospective studies. In a first work including 49 infants with a mean gestational age 30.9 ± 2.7 weeks (range 25–35 weeks), neonates with any stage of retinopathy of prematurity (ROP) had higher HbA and lower HbF levels at postnatal months 1 and 2 compared with those without ROP.[20] However, the analysis of covariance that ignored transfusions revealed no difference between the means of Hb variants in patients with and without ROP. Indeed, the authors concluded that RBC transfusion significantly reduced HbF in premature infants, whereas HbF/HbA had no direct effect on the development of ROP.[20] In a subsequent study including 42 preterm neonates (mean gestation 28.0 weeks, SD 1.91),

Stutchfield and colleagues reported that HbF levels during hospitalization were significantly lower in infants with any stage of ROP in comparison to neonates without ROP (61.7 vs 91.9%, $P = .0001$).[21] Overall, there was a strong association between mean HbF and increasing ROP severity.[21] The PacIFiHER trial, which included 60 neonates with gestational age less than 31 weeks, concluded that mean HbF levels at 31 and 34 postconceptional weeks were associated with an increased risk for mild or severe ROP.[22] Similar conclusions were reached by Hellström and colleagues in a retrospective series of 452 infants (mean gestational age 26.4 ± 1.7 weeks): neonates developing any stage of ROP had equivalent HbF at birth but lower HbF levels after the first postnatal week.[23] A higher fraction of HbF during the first postnatal week was associated with a lower prevalence of any ROP (with an OR of 0.83 by a 10% HbF increase, 95% CI: 0.71–0.97) and of severe ROP.[23] In the same series of neonates, lower levels of HbF during the first postnatal week were also associated with an increased risk for bronchopulmonary dysplasia (BPD).[24] This finding confirmed previous observations reported by Perrone and colleagues in a smaller series of patients.[25]

IS FETAL HEMOGLOBIN PROTECTIVE IN PRETERM NEONATES?

The studies mentioned above suggest that the early HbF loss and the consequent exposure to HbA may convey an additional risk for developing prematurity-related comorbidities, as ROP or BPD. However, although the Hb switch is largely genetically regulated, it has been reported that HbF levels may increase in the perinatal period as a compensatory mechanism for hypoxemia and anemia.[26,27] It is therefore conceivable that high-HbF levels in premature infants may play a role even after birth, exerting a protective effect during their complicated clinical course.

The oxidative stress is the pathophysiological driver of preterm neonate frailty.[28] Given their immature antioxidant defense, it has been suggested that the abnormal amount of oxygen released from HbA may represent a hyperoxic challenge to developing organs.[29] It has been shown that in patients with hemoglobinopathies the oxygen volume released at level of peripheral tissues may vary up of 50% depending on the 2,3 BPG concentration and hemoglobin oxygen affinity.[30] In these adult patients, reducing Hb oxygen affinity to increase oxygen delivery is a compensatory mechanism to alleviate the effects of anemia. On the opposite, in preterm neonates, the increased oxygen delivery from high HbA may result at cellular level in a dangerous condition of hyperoxia, with consequent overproduction of reactive oxygen species (ROS).[31] In the context of a hyperoxic situation, cellular survival depends on the antioxidant defenses to counteract the effects of ROS.[31] Unfortunately, in preterm neonates, antioxidant resources to harness the hyperoxic burden are deeply insufficient.[28] Notably, data gathered in the PacIFiHER study clearly demonstrated that lower levels of HbF are associated with poorer indices of systemic oxygenation, as measured by median levels of peripheral oxygen saturation and partial pressure of carbon dioxide.[32] The authors proposed that the better oxygenation in neonates with high-HbF levels could be due to the higher HbF capacity to carry oxygen, with the Bohr effect at peripheral tissue level exceeding the high oxygen affinity.[32] In addition, we could also hypothesize that, under an initial hypoxia condition, microcirculatory blood flow might be better regulated and preserved by HbF than HbA, with low-HbF levels further exacerbating the impaired oxygenation through a poor tissue perfusion. Although this assumption is merely speculative, several evidence exist that bioactive NO availability is higher with higher HbF levels. For example, higher SNO-HbF levels have been demonstrated in preterm neonates with gestational age less than 30 weeks compared with infants aged 30 weeks or older.[33] Moreover, faster oxidative denitrosylation and more efficient transfer of bioactive NO for HbF than HbA have been documented in in vitro and in vivo experimental models.[34,35] An additional reason accounting for a better perfusion in the presence of high HbF is the superior deformability of neonatal RBCs in comparison with adult RBCs.[36] Notably, RBC with poorer deformability induces lower capillary recruitment, which results in the reduced tissue oxygenation.[37] RBC deformability is also a reliable indicator of the hemolysis propensity of RBCs and correlates with the hemolysis rate during the blood product storage.[38] In patients with thalassemia receiving transfusions, RBC deformability correlates with plasma free hemoglobin, transfusion efficiency, and microcirculation blood flow.[39,40] In patients with sickle cell disease, there is an inverse and significant correlation between percentage of HbF and RBC deformability, suggesting that a high-HbF content can improve erythrocytes hydration and deformability.[41]

The HbF molecule is endowed with a robust structural stability, allowing to maintain the tetrameric integrity, which probably explains its evolutionary advantage.[42,43] This characteristic seems to be relevant almost if hemoglobin spreads to the extracellular environment. Free hemoglobin affects redox status and mitochondrial dynamic of surrounding cells and tissues, and elicits a wide range of biological reactions, including inflammatory response and proliferation.[44] Various studies have shown that, in comparison with HbA, HbF exhibits slower rates of heme loss, heme-derived iron release, and lower proficiency to the DNA cleavage.[43,45] HbF is also endowed with a higher intrinsic pseudoperoxidase activity.[46] These characteristics, on the one hand reduce oxidative burden and cell membrane injury due to lipid peroxidation, and, on the other hand, neutralize peroxides and remove radicals through a peroxide radical-self termination reaction that generates more stable molecules.[46,47]

Finally, it is worth to emphasize that the HbF decrease may have a different influence depending on several patient and disease-related concurrent variables. Indeed, the influence of a severe HbF reduction might be different in patients receiving or not oxygen therapy. Moreover, transfusions at different ages may have a different influence on specific organ or tissues: for example, the period in which RBC transfusions interfere with retinal vascularization may be critical for ROP increase and progression. Accordingly, severe ROP has been associated with either RBC transfusion in the first 10 days of life or with receiving 2 or more RBC transfusions within the postconceptional age of 29 weeks.[23,48,49]

CORD BLOOD TRANSFUSION PREVENTS FETAL HEMOGLOBIN LOSS

All strategies delaying and/or reducing transfusion requirements in preterm neonates are potentially able to limit the HbF loss or postpone it at later development stages, less prone to be affected from the HbF deficiency. These strategies are widely applicable and include delayed cord clamping, stringent indications for blood sampling, adoption of point-of-care testing with minimal sample volumes, or tight adherence to recommended Hb thresholds for transfusion.[50] Particularly if collectively adopted, these measures are reasonably able to limit transfusion needs of preterm neonates, so restraining the HbF depletion. Our group has been working on an additional strategy, setting an alternative transfusion approach based on allogeneic RBC concentrates obtained from CB of full-term neonates. Umbilical CB has been used for pediatric transfusion in different clinical settings.[51] In neonatal transfusion, autologous CB has been used when surgery was planned before the delivery for congenital heart diseases.[51] Extremely premature neonates, however, require repeated transfusions over a prolonged period, so that autologous transfusion is impracticable. We, therefore, set an automated processing method to recover RBC concentrates from

CB units donated at our public CB bank.[52] A great proportion of units usually collected at public CB banks are otherwise suitable for transplant but have a low nucleated cell content, prompting their utilization as source material for alternative uses.[53] For manufacturing CB RBC concentrates, we adopted the same quality standards as for standard RBC products: hematocrit value between 50% and 70%, residual white blood cells after filtration less than 1×10^6, and percentage of hemolysis at the end of the storage less than 0.8%.[54] In addition to standard infectious disease tests, cultures for bacterial and fungal contamination are regularly performed.[52] CB RBC units are suspended in Saline, Adenine, Glucose-mannitol, stored at $4 \pm 2°C$ for a maximum of 14 days to allow γ-irradiation.[52] We carried out a first feasibility study, including newborns with gestational age of 30 weeks or lesser and/or birth weight of 1500 g or greater.[55] At first transfusion, patients were assigned to receive CB RBCs or adult RBCs depending on the availability of ABO-Rh(D)-matched CB RBC units; the same product type was assigned (if available) in the subsequent transfusion events. A total of 20 patients were included and a total of 23 CB were transfused to 9 patients. No acute or delayed transfusion-related adverse events were recorded. **Table 1** displays hematocrit and biochemical parameters recorded in patients participating to the study, before and after CB or standard transfusions.[55] Subsequently, we performed a "proof of concept" study to demonstrate that CB RBC units can prevent the HbF depletion in transfused neonates.[19] Twenty-five neonates with gestational age less than 30 weeks were enrolled, and HbF levels were recorded until 36 weeks of postmenstrual age (PMA). Patients received RBC units from CB or adult donors depending on whether compatible CB RBCs were available. Primary outcome was HbF level at PMA of 32 weeks. At 32 and 36 weeks of PMA, HbF levels were significantly higher in neonates transfused with CB RBCs than in neonates receiving adult RBCs or both RBC types. **Fig. 1** shows the HbF values plotted against PMA, recorded in enrolled patients: values are grouped according to the transfusion types received at the time of HbF recording.[19] Whereas patients with ROP and BPD had HbF values in the lowest quartile, the study was not designed to investigate clinical effects and could not reliably assess if higher HbF percentages also reduced the occurrence and severity of these diseases.[19]

Table 1
Biochemical parameters before and after transfusing RBC concentrates obtained from umbilical blood or adult donors. Data are relative to patients enrolled in the study reported in reference n.55

	Cord RBCs (n = 23)	P value	Adult RBCs (n = 27)	P value
Transfused RBC (mL/kg)[a]	19.8 ± 1.16		20.1 ± 1.2	
Hct pre (%)	31.1 ± 2.5	<.001	31.9 ± 3.3	<.001
Hct post (%)	43.1 ± 5.0		44.8 ± 5.2	
Glucose pre (mg/dL)	116.8 ± 49.5	.363	109.3 ± 44.2	.459
Glucose post (mg/dL)	103.8 ± 41.5		115.9 ± 50.1	
pH pre	7.28 ± 0.07	.571	7.27 ± 0.06	.726
pH post	7.29 ± 0.07		7.27 ± 0.09	
K pre (mmol/L)	4.1 ± 0.8	.527	4.6 ± 0.7	.581
K post (mmol/L)	4.2 ± 0.8		4.6 ± 0.8	
Lactate pre (mmol/L)	1.9 ± 1.9	.573	1.9 ± 1.7	.047
Lactate post (mmol/L)	1.6 ± 1.5		1.4 ± 0.9	

[a] Transfusion doses were similar between groups: $P = .965$ at Mann Whitney test.

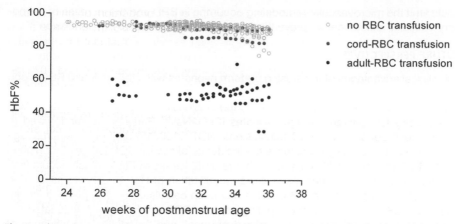

Fig. 1. HbF values recorded in patients participating to the CB-Trip study (reference n.19). Data are expressed as percentage of total hemoglobin and are plotted against the PMA at testing. Values are grouped according to transfusion types (no transfusion, cord blood transfusions, and adult donor transfusions).

Cord Blood Transfusions and Prematurity Diseases

The postnatal oxidative stress is the main driver of pathologic conditions connected to the premature birth.[56] During their clinical course, preterm infants, who are naturally endowed with an immature antioxidant system, experience several situations prompting the production of free radicals, including resuscitative maneuvers and mechanical ventilation, surfactant administration, parenteral nutrition, infections, or blood product transfusion.[57] In addition, preterm infants are frequently exposed to improper partial oxygen tensions.[57] Finally, these patients are at risk of free-iron accumulation derived from hemolysis following intraventricular hemorrhage, or from free-iron increase in erythrocytes in consequence of asphyxia or acidosis, resulting in membrane protein oxidation, and free iron release into the plasma.[58–60] As previously reported, a clear association between ROP and low-HbF levels has been found in retrospective and prospective studies.[21–23] Moreover, ROP has been related to both the number of blood products and age at transfusions.[61] ROP has a multifactorial pathogenesis, encompassing several risk factors occurring during intrauterine and postnatal life.[62] Among them, the premature exposure to high-oxygen concentrations can trigger an initial growth arrest of retinal vessels through the overproduction of ROS, inflammatory activation, damage of vascular endothelial cells, and microvascular degeneration. After the initial suppression of angiogenesis, the angio-proliferative phase is triggered by the compensatory release of proangiogenic factors, vascular endothelial growth factor, and the progressive increase of insulin-like growth factor-1.[62] The association between low-HbF levels and BPD has also been reported.[24,25] Mechanisms responsible for BPD include hyperoxia that causes the release of ROS, cell death, inhibition of the alveolarization, inflammation, and impaired pulmonary angiogenesis.[63,64] The oxidative stress induced by hyperoxia perturbs normal differentiation and survival of alveolar epithelial type-II cells, the most important stem cells in lung tissue responsible for functioning and postinjury repair of alveolar epithelial structures.[65] In both ROP and BPD, physiologic HbF levels could exert a protective effect through a smoother oxygen release, limiting the hyperoxia damaging effect. Moreover, improving the regulation of microcirculatory blood flow through a more efficient NO delivery, HbF could have a favorable effect also on the abnormal vessel proliferation. In particular, HbF could limit the microvascular remodeling occurring in BPD and the increase of pulmonary vascular resistance, so preventing or attenuating pulmonary hypertension.[66]

FUTURE PERSPECTIVES

The clinical advantages of transfusing preterm neonates with HbF-enriched RBC blood products remain speculative and need to be demonstrated. The multicenter randomized trial BORN is ongoing to assess if CB RBC transfusions can reduce the severity of ROP in extremely low gestational age neonates (ELGANs).[67] Patients are randomized to receive adult donor or CB RBC transfusions (NCT05100212) until postmenstrual age of 32 weeks. The primary outcome is the incidence of severe ROP (stages 3 or higher) in CB RBC and adult RBC arms at discharge or 40 weeks of PMA, which occurs first. Among secondary outcomes, there is the identification of HbF thresholds associated with ROP. A sample size of 146 patients has been calculated, with a planned interim analysis at 58 patients. In all participating centers, RBC products are fractionated according to a semiautomated standardized protocol, and to validate the influence of the storage length, the data relative to the quality of all produced units are collected in parallel with clinical enrollment. An additional pilot, open label, nonrandomized, single-center study on CB transfusion in preterm neonates is registered at ClinicalTrial.gov (NCT05612919). The main objective is to evaluate the safety, feasibility, and efficacy of CB RBC transfusion in extremely preterm infants. A sample size of 30 patients is reported. At the time of writing the study was not yet recruiting.

SUMMARY

The growing interest on the use of CB RBC for transfusing preterm neonates is, in part, explained by the prospective to recycle many CB units otherwise destined to disposal.[68,69] In this regard, however, it is worth to mention that processing CB into RBC concentrates is time-consuming and has additional costs in terms of personnel, consumables, and microbial testing. Many technical aspects are still to be defined. For example, it could be worth to introduce nucleic acid screening for microbial contaminants, to shorten the interval between production and release. Moreover, implementing the CB transfusion program for preterm neonates would imply a close cooperation among blood banks serving neonatal intensive care units and CB banks. A CB-centered transfusion network should be designed, identifying specific logistic frames, technical agreements, and transport arrangements. Therefore, a dedicated health technology assessment analyzing all the above-mentioned aspects is encouraged, to better clarify the economic impact of a wide realization of this transfusion strategy. Hopefully, the evidence of clinical advantages of transfusing preterm neonates with CB RBC concentrates will prompt to find solutions for the aforesaid drawbacks.

Finally, it would be desirable that clinical data of patients receiving CB transfusions are complemented by the exploration of oxidative stress biomarkers, as well by regional tissue oxygenation monitoring through near infrared spectroscopy. This could allow to understand the biological basis of the putative protective effect exerted by allogeneic RBC transfusion.

Best Practices Box

What is the current practice for transfusion therapy for ELGANs?

Current Practice: RBC concentrates routinely used for transfusion therapy for prematurity anemia are obtained from adult donors. Repeated RBC transfusions produce in preterm neonates the progressive replacement of HbF by HbA.

What changes in current practice are likely to improve outcomes?

HbA, with lower oxygen affinity, may result in higher oxygen delivery and exacerbation of the oxidative burden. This could explain the association between RBC transfusions and diseases related to oxidative damage, such as retinopathy or BPD. Notably, the antioxidant response in ELGANs is highly immature and inadequate to manage oxidative challenges. Transfusing ELGANs with RBC obtained from allogeneic CB increases hemoglobin levels without depleting HbF. Moreover, this approach could preserve the physiologic oxygen delivery to developing organs and tissues.

Pearls/Pitfalls: CB-RBC transfusion is an effective strategy to prevent the HbF depletion due to repeated transfusions. The beneficial effect of this approach in limiting the severity of diseases correlated to oxidative damage is to be demonstrated.

Major recommendations

- Future trials evaluating morbidity and mortality in ELGANs receiving standard or CB-RBC transfusion are warranted.

Bibliographic Source(s)

- Stutchfield CJ, Jain A, Odd D, Williams C, Markham R. Fetal hemoglobin, blood transfusion, and retinopathy of prematurity in very preterm infants: a pilot prospective cohort study. Eye (Lond). 2017;31(10):1451 to 1455. https://doi.org/10.1038/eye.2017.76.
- Hellström W, Martinsson T, Hellstrom A, Morsing E, Ley D. Fetal hemoglobin and bronchopulmonary dysplasia in neonates: an observational study. Arch Dis Child Fetal Neonatal Ed. 2021;106(1):88 to 92. https://doi.org/10.1136/archdischild-2020-319181.
- Teofili L, Papacci P, Orlando N, Bianchi M, Molisso A, Purcaro V, Valentini CG, Giannantonio C, Serrao F, Chiusolo P, Nicolotti N, Pellegrino C, Carducci B, Vento G, De Stefano V. Allogeneic cord blood transfusions prevent fetal hemoglobin depletion in preterm neonates. Results of the CB-TrIP study. Br J Haematol. 2020;191(2):263 to 268. doi: 10.1111/bjh.16851.

DISCLOSURE

The authors have no financial interests to disclose.

REFERENCES

1. Wood WG, Weatherall DJ. Haemoglobin synthesis during human foetal development. Nature 1973;244(5412):162–5.
2. Bard H. The postnatal decline of hemoglobin F synthesis in normal full-term infants. J Clin Invest 1975;55(2):395–8.
3. Bard H. Postnatal fetal and adult hemoglobin synthesis in early preterm newborn infants. J Clin Invest 1973;52(8):1789–95.
4. Bou-Fakhredin R, De Franceschi L, Motta I, et al. Pharmacological induction of fetal hemoglobin in β-thalassemia and sickle cell disease: an updated perspective. Pharmaceuticals 2022;15(6):753.
5. Sankaran VG, Menne TF, Xu J, et al. Human fetal hemoglobin expression is regulated by the developmental stage-specific repressor BCL11A. Science 2008; 322(5909):1839–42.
6. Huang P, Peslak SA, Ren R, et al. HIC2 controls developmental hemoglobin switching by repressing BCL11A transcription. Nat Genet 2022;54(9):1417–26.
7. Adachi K, Konitzer P, Pang J, et al. Amino acids responsible for decreased 2,3-biphosphoglycerate binding to fetal hemoglobin. Blood 1997;90(8):2916–20.
8. Ruan B, Paulson RF. Metabolic regulation of stress erythropoiesis, outstanding questions, and possible paradigms. Front Physiol 2023;13:1063294.

9. Feng R, Mayuranathan T, Huang P, et al. Activation of γ-globin expression by hypoxia-inducible factor 1α. Nature 2022;610(7933):783–90.

10. Grubina R, Huang Z, Shiva S, et al. Concerted nitric oxide formation and release from the simultaneous reactions of nitrite with deoxy- and oxyhemoglobin. J Biol Chem 2007;282(17):12916–27.

11. Zhang R, Hess DT, Qian Z, et al. Hemoglobin βCys93 is essential for cardiovascular function and integrated response to hypoxia. Proc Natl Acad Sci U S A 2015;112(20):6425–30.

12. Isbell TS, Sun CW, Wu LC, et al. SNO-hemoglobin is not essential for red blood cell-dependent hypoxic vasodilation. Nat Med 2008;14(7):773–7.

13. Reynolds JD, Posina K, Zhu L, et al. Control of tissue oxygenation by S-nitroso-hemoglobin in human subjects. Proc Natl Acad Sci U S A 2023;120(9). e2220769120.

14. Zhang R, Hausladen A, Qian Z, et al. Hypoxic vasodilatory defect and pulmonary hypertension in mice lacking hemoglobin β-cysteine93 S-nitrosylation. JCI Insight 2022;7(3):e155234.

15. De Halleux V, Truttmann A, Gagnon C, et al. The effect of blood transfusion on the hemoglobin oxygen dissociation curve of very early preterm infants during the first week of life. Semin Perinatol 2002;26(6):411–5.

16. Watanabe Y, Osawa K, Sato I, et al. Foetal haemoglobin concentration at post-menstrual age is unaffected by gestational age at birth. Ann Clin Biochem 2018;55(3):400–3.

17. Gavulic AE, Dougherty D, Li SH, et al. Fetal hemoglobin levels in premature new-borns. Should we reconsider transfusion of adult donor blood? J Pediatr Surg 2021;56(11):1944–8.

18. Bednarczuk N, Williams EE, Kaltsogianni O, et al. Postnatal temporal changes of foetal haemoglobin in prematurely born infants. Acta Paediatr 2022;111(7): 1338–40.

19. Teofili L, Papacci P, Orlando N, et al. Allogeneic cord blood transfusions prevent fetal haemoglobin depletion in preterm neonates. Results of the CB-TrIP study. Br J Haematol 2020;191(2):263–8.

20. Erdol H, Hacioglu D, Kola M, et al. Investigation of the effect of hemoglobin F and A levels on development of retinopathy of prematurity. J AAPOS 2017;21(2): 136–40.

21. Stutchfield CJ, Jain A, Odd D, et al. Foetal haemoglobin, blood transfusion, and retinopathy of prematurity in very preterm infants: a pilot prospective cohort study. Eye (Lond). 2017;31(10):1451–5.

22. Jiramongkolchai K, Repka MX, Tian J, et al. Lower foetal haemoglobin levels at 31- and 34-weeks post menstrual age is associated with the development of retinopathy of prematurity : PacIFiHER Report No. 1 PacIFiHER Study Group (Preterm Infants and Fetal Haemoglobin in ROP). Eye (Lond). 2021;35(2):659–64.

23. Hellström W, Martinsson T, Morsing E, et al. Low fraction of fetal haemoglobin is associated with retinopathy of prematurity in the very preterm infant. Br J Ophthalmol 2022;106(7):970–4.

24. Hellstrom W, Martinsson T, Hellstrom A, et al. Fetal haemoglobin and bronchopulmonary dysplasia in neonates: an observational study. Arch Dis Child Fetal Neonatal Ed 2021;106(1):88–92.

25. Perrone B, Marchionni P, Bartoli A, et al. 258 fetal haemoglobin levels in preterm infants at 36 Weeks postmenstrual age: effect of bronchopulmonary dysplasia. Sepsis and Transfusions Archives of Disease in Childhood 2012;97:A75.

26. Bard H. Hypoxemia and increased fetal hemoglobin synthesis during the peri-natal period. Semin Perinatol 1992;16:191–5.

27. Bard H, Lachance C, Widness JA, et al. The reactivation of fetal hemoglobin synthesis during anemia of prematurity. Pediatr Res 1994;36:253–6.

28. Moore TA, Ahmad IM, Zimmerman MC. Oxidative stress and preterm birth: an integrative review. Biol Res Nurs 2018;20(5):497–512.

29. Podraza W. A new approach to neonatal medical management that could transform the prevention of retinopathy of prematurity: theoretical considerations. Med Hypotheses 2020;137:109541.

30. Bunn HF. Oxygen delivery in the treatment of anemia. N Engl J Med 2022; 387(25):2362–5.

31. Tretter V, Zach ML, Bohme S, et al. Investigating disturbances of oxygen homeostasis: from cellular mechanisms to the clinical practice. Front Physiol 2020; 11:947.

32. Jiramongkolchai K, Repka MX, Tian J, et al. PacIFiHER study group (preterm infants and foetal haemoglobin in retinopathy of prematurity). Effects of fetal haemoglobin on systemic oxygenation in preterm infants and the development of retinopathy of prematurity PacIFiHER Report No. 2. Br J Ophthalmol 2023; 107(3):380–3.

33. Riccio DA, Malowitz JR, Cotten CM, et al. S-Nitrosylated fetal hemoglobin in neonatal human blood. Biochem Biophys Res Commun 2016;473(4):1084–9.

34. Blood AB, Tiso M, Verma ST, et al. Increased nitrite reductase activity of fetal versus adult ovine hemoglobin. Am J Physiol Heart Circ Physiol 2009;296(2): H237–46.

35. Salhany JM. The oxidative denitrosylation mechanism and nitric oxide release from human fetal and adult hemoglobin, an experimentally based model simulation study. Blood Cells Mol Dis 2013;50(1):8–19.

36. Arbell D, Bin-Nun A, Zugayar D, et al. Deformability of cord blood vs. newborns' red blood cells: implication for blood transfusion. J Matern Fetal Neonatal Med 2022;35(17):3270–5.

37. Parthasarathi K, Lipowsky HH. Capillary recruitment in response to tissue hypoxia and its dependence on red blood cell deformability. Am J Physiol 1999;277(6): H2145–57.

38. Relevy H, Koshkaryev A, Manny N, et al. Blood banking-induced alteration of red blood cell flow properties. Transfusion 2008;48(1):136–46.

39. Barshtein G, Goldschmidt N, Pries AR, et al. Deformability of transfused red blood cells is a potent effector of transfusion-induced hemoglobin increment: a study with β-thalassemia major patients. Am J Hematol 2017;92(9):E559–60.

40. Barshtein G, Pries AR, Goldschmidt N, et al. Deformability of transfused red blood cells is a potent determinant of transfusion-induced change in recipient's blood flow. Microcirculation 2016;23(7):479–86.

41. Parrow NL, Tu H, Nichols J, et al. Measurements of red cell deformability and hydration reflect HbF and HbA2 in blood from patients with sickle cell anemia. Blood Cells Mol Dis 2017;65:41–50.

42. Reeder BJ. The redox activity of hemoglobins: from physiologic functions to pathologic mechanisms. Antioxid Redox Signal 2010;13(7):1087–123.

43. Simons M, Gretton S, Silkstone GGA, et al. Comparison of the oxidative reactivity of recombinant fetal and adult human hemoglobin: implications for the design of hemoglobin-based oxygen carriers. Biosci Rep 2018;38(4). BSR20180370.

44. Drvenica IT, Stancic AZ, Maslovaric IS, et al. Extracellular hemoglobin: modulation of cellular functions and pathophysiological effects. Biomolecules 2022; 12(11):1708.
45. Chakane S, Matos T, Kettisen K, et al. Fetal hemoglobin is much less prone to DNA cleavage compared to the adult protein. Redox Biol 2017;12:114–20.
46. Ratanasopa K, Strader MB, Alayash AI, et al. Dissection of the radical reactions linked to fetal hemoglobin reveals enhanced pseudoperoxidase activity. Front Physiol 2015;6:39.
47. Chiabrando D, Vinchi F, Fiorito V, et al. Heme in pathophysiology: a matter of scavenging, metabolism and trafficking across cell membranes. Front Pharmacol 2014;5:61.
48. Lust C, Vesoulis Z, Jackups R, et al. Early red cell transfusion is associated with development of severe retinopathy of prematurity. J Perinatol 2019;39(3): 393–400.
49. Teofili L, Papacci P, Bartolo M, et al. Transfusion-free survival predicts severe retinopathy in preterm neonates. Front Pediatr 2022;10:814194.
50. Saito-Benz M, Flanagan P, Berry MJ. Management of anaemia in pre-term infants. Br J Haematol 2020;188(3):354–66.
51. Bianchi M, Papacci P, Valentini CG, et al. Umbilical cord blood as a source for red-blood-cell transfusion in neonatology: a systematic review. Vox Sang 2018; 113(8):713–25.
52. Bianchi M, Orlando N, Barbagallo O, et al. Allogeneic cord blood red blood cells: assessing cord blood unit fractionation and validation. Blood Transfus 2021; 19(5):435–44.
53. Querol S, Rubinstein P, Madrigal A. The wider perspective: cord blood banks and their future prospects. Br J Haematol 2021;195(4):507–17.
54. European Directorate for the Quality of Medicines & HealthCare. European Committee on Blood Transfusion. Guide to the preparation, use and quality assurance of blood components. 20th edition. (last accessed March 30, 2023) Available at https://www.edqm.eu/en/blood-guide
55. Bianchi M, Giannantonio C, Spartano S, et al. Allogeneic umbilical cord blood red cell concentrates: an innovative blood product for transfusion therapy of preterm infants. Neonatology 2015;107(2):81–6.
56. Perez M, Robbins ME, Revhaug C, et al. Oxygen radical disease in the newborn, revisited: oxidative stress and disease in the newborn period. Free Radic Biol Med 2019;142:61–72.
57. Lembo C, Buonocore G, Perrone S. Oxidative stress in preterm newborns. Antioxidants 2021;10(11):1672.
58. Ciccoli L, Rossi V, Leoncini S, et al. Iron release in erythrocytes and plasma non protein-bound iron in hypoxic and non hypoxic newborns. Free Radic Res 2003; 37(1):51–8.
59. Agyemang AA, Kvist SV, Brinkman N, et al. Cell-free oxidized hemoglobin drives reactive oxygen species production and pro-inflammation in an immature primary rat mixed glial cell culture. J Neuroinflammation 2021;18(1):42.
60. Perrone S, Laschi E, Buonocore G. Biomarkers of oxidative stress in the fetus and in the newborn. Free Radic Biol Med 2019;142:23–31.
61. Hengartner T, Adams M, Pfister RE, et al, Swiss Neonatal Network. Associations between red blood cell and platelet transfusions and retinopathy of prematurity. Neonatology 2020;117(5):1–7.
62. Hellstrom A, Smith LE, Dammann O. Retinopathy of prematurity. Lancet 2013; 382(9902):1445–57.

63. Perrone S, Tataranno ML, Buonocore G. Oxidative stress and bronchopulmonary dysplasia. J Clin Neonatol 2012;1(3):109–14.
64. Kimble A, Robbins ME, Perez M. Pathogenesis of bronchopulmonary dysplasia: role of oxidative stress from 'Omics' studies. Antioxidants 2022;11(12):2380.
65. Hou A, Fu J, Yang H, et al. Hyperoxia stimulates the transdifferentiation of type II alveolar epithelial cells in newborn rats. Am J Physiol Lung Cell Mol Physiol 2015; 308(9):L861–72.
66. Alvira CM. Aberrant pulmonary vascular growth and remodeling in bronchopulmonary dysplasia. Front Med 2016;3:21.
67. Teofili L, Papacci P, Orlando N, et al. BORN study: a multicenter randomized trial investigating cord blood red blood cell transfusions to reduce the severity of retinopathy of prematurity in extremely low gestational age neonates. Trials 2022; 23(1):1010.
68. Gonzalez EG, Casanova MA, Samarkanova D, et al. Feasibility of umbilical cord blood as a source of red blood cell transfusion in preterm infants. Blood Transfus 2021;19(6):510–7.
69. Rebulla P, Querol S, Pupella S, et al. Recycling apparent waste into biologicals: the case of umbilical cord blood in Italy and Spain. Front Cell Dev Biol 2022;9: 812038.

Near-Infrared Spectroscopy to Guide and Understand Effects of Red Blood Cell Transfusion

Sean M. Bailey, MD*, Pradeep V. Mally, MD

KEYWORDS

- Near-infrared spectroscopy • Regional tissue oxygen saturation
- Fractional tissue oxygen extraction • Blood transfusion

KEY POINTS

- There is variability in current neonatal red blood cell (RBC) transfusion practices.
- Traditional markers indicating a transfusion is necessary, namely hemoglobin and hematocrit, may be too generalizable and nonspecific for a highly variable neonatal population.
- Near-infrared spectroscopy (NIRS) has been shown capable of demonstrating changes that occur in tissue oxygenation levels resulting from an RBC transfusion in neonates.
- However, it has not yet been demonstrated by clinical researchers exactly how NIRS can be used to specifically guide transfusion practice.
- Further studies and analysis are needed to determine if NIRS can be fully incorporated into a blood transfusion management strategy.

INTRODUCTION

The use of red blood cell (RBC) transfusion in the neonatal intensive care unit (NICU) setting is commonplace and remains an important therapeutic intervention.[1] This is especially the case during the care of preterm infants who are often hospitalized in the NICU for months.[2] In fact, it has been reported that the patient population with extremely low birth weight (ELBW) is likely exposed to more RBC transfusions than almost any other group, with a vast majority receiving a transfusion during their NICU course, and often multiple times.[3]

In recent years, there has been increasing analysis and scrutiny concerning the amount of RBC transfusions occurring in the NICU setting.[4] Current prevailing thought among neonatologists is that perhaps so many transfusions could be doing more

Division of Neonatology, Department of Pediatrics, NYU Grossman School of Medicine, Hassenfeld Children's Hospital NYU Langone, 317 East 34th Street, Suite 902, New York, NY 10016, USA
* Corresponding author. NYU Division of Neonatology, 317 East 34th Street, Suite 902, New York, NY 10016.
E-mail address: sean.bailey@nyulangone.org

Clin Perinatol 50 (2023) 895–910
https://doi.org/10.1016/j.clp.2023.07.006
0095-5108/23/© 2023 Elsevier Inc. All rights reserved.

perinatology.theclinics.com

harm than good.[5] Or, at the very least, there is a belief that administration of more RBC transfusions may not improve outcomes in most cases.[6] This belief primarily comes from several studies demonstrating that using liberal RBC transfusion guidelines add no more benefit to neonatal patients' short-term or long-term outcomes than using restrictive transfusion practices.[7,8] In addition, neonatal physicians often consider the numerous studies suggesting that RBC transfusion could have potential deleterious consequences.[9] This includes multiple complications encountered in the NICU that might be associated with RBC transfusion, including necrotizing enterocolitis, retinopathy of prematurity, intraventricular hemorrhage, and lung injury.[10–13]

Regardless of a clinician's exact RBC transfusion practice tendencies, they continue to rely on hemoglobin (Hgb) or hematocrit (HCT) as the primary marker that would trigger transfusion.[14] However, neither Hgb nor HCT may actually reflect the true transfusion needs of an individual neonate, especially in patients with ELBW that often are experiencing anemia of prematurity and are able to compensate.[15] Neonatologists increasingly recognize that a Hgb level that may be inadequate to meet the oxygen carrying capacity needs for one infant might be perfectly fine for another; all depending on the specific metabolic demands and oxygen supply requirements of a patient at a given point in time.[16] Therefore, clinical researchers are continuously evaluating for new markers that may more accurately reflect transfusion need.[17] This search has included the use of ultrasound techniques to assess cardiac output and tissue perfusion indices, assessment of serum lactate levels, monitoring for intermittent hypoxia, as well as measuring tissue oxygen saturation levels with near-infrared spectroscopy (NIRS) devices.[18–21] This review will focus on the use of NIRS and its place in helping to better understand and define neonatal anemia, determine the physiologic changes that transpire when infants receive RBC transfusions, and understand how NIRS could help guide transfusion management in the NICU.

CURRENT RED BLOOD CELL TRANSFUSION PRACTICES IN NEONATES

At present, Hgb or HCT are by far the most common objective parameters that NICU transfusion guidelines are based on.[22] These values are derived from predetermined normal levels and are used to recommend intervention.[23] Many protocols also consider either a neonate's gestational age or day of life, along with intensity of respiratory support, with the aim of improving predictability of RBC transfusion success.[24] Clinicians in the NICU might also consider other comorbidities, degree of clinical stability, growth status, and reticulocyte count when making a transfusion determination.[25] Based on the clinical data they have at hand, along with transfusion guideline resources available to them, a physician or clinical team can then decide to either order an RBC transfusion or continue observation. It is important to note that many guidelines also suggest that clinical judgment should be considered.

Variation in neonatal RBC transfusion practice exists because (1) there are no universally accepted published guidelines, (2) unit specific algorithms can vary, and (3) clinical judgment differs among clinicians based on previous experiences and altering opinions.[26] This is supported by evidence from international surveys demonstrating a very wide variation in practice and differing Hgb/HCT parameters likely used to trigger neonatal transfusion.[27] It has also been shown that even within major US academic medical centers, neonatal RBC transfusion practices can often vary.[28]

Although following stricter laboratory value-based guidelines, there can still exist much variation in the number of RBC transfusions that neonates are exposed to. This is best exemplified by the fact that in the 2 most recent large neonatal transfusion trials, the Transfusion of Prematures (TOP) trial and the Effects of Transfusion

Thresholds on Neurocognitive Outcomes (ETTNO)study, there were significant differences found in the number of RBC transfusions that subjects received between studies.[29] This is despite very similar study subject demographics and transfusion triggers.[7,8]

Neonatal care teams are now not just developing specific guidelines that are clear and easily accessible but are also stressing that physicians should pause and think carefully about parameters and clinical indications before ordering an RBC transfusion.[30] However, even with all of the latest evidence and best of intentions, this does not always translate into universally decreasing RBC transfusions in the NICU, and much heterogeneity in care can occur.[31] There then clearly exists a need to find a new transfusion marker, or an adjunctive one, that could help decrease unnecessary transfusions using physiologic data in individual patients. This is where the thought process of using NIRS in transfusion practice originated.

Basis for and History of Near-Infrared Spectroscopy Use in Neonatal Clinical Care

The application of near-infrared light to monitor oxygen saturation (SaO_2) levels has long been used in medicine. This is possible based on 3 primary principles: (1) tissue is relatively transparent to light in the near-infrared range, (2) oxygenated Hgb and deoxygenated Hgb are the main chromophores that absorb light at this spectrum, and (3) they both have their own light absorption properties.[32] Therefore, by directing light at these wavelengths to penetrate the skin using emitters, detection sensors can subsequently determine the amount or percent of oxygenated Hgb that exists in comparison to the total amount of Hgb present.

Pulse oximetry, a well-established and almost universally applied monitoring modality, uses near-infrared light in this manner to determine the SaO_2 of arterial blood. NIRS incorporates similar techniques but the light emitters penetrate somewhat deeper into tissue where organs lie and the detectors placed over various organs (ie, brain, kidney, and gut) are able to then determine the percent of oxygenated Hgb in the tissue below

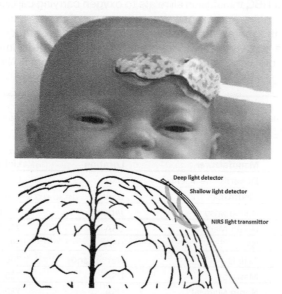

Fig. 1. A NIRS sensor monitoring $CrSO_2$ and corresponding graphic demonstrating near-infrared light penetrating skull in order to measure brain tissue values.

compared with total Hgb[33] (see **Fig. 1**). The blood supply in the area that NIRS is monitoring, in contrast to pulse oximetry, is made up of a blood vessel mixture, including the arterial, capillary, and venous microcirculation. The value that NIRS provides is known as regional tissue oxygen saturation (rSO_2). Therefore, although SaO_2 essentially only provides information about the blood oxygen supply, rSO_2 can provide clinicians with information about the balance between tissue blood supply in comparison to tissue demand. In addition, clinicians can use SaO_2 data along with rSO_2 data to calculate a fractional tissue oxygen extraction (FTOE) value of organ tissue using the following formula: $FTOE = (SaO_2 - rSO_2)/SaO_2$. The FTOE gives an indication of how much oxygen is being extracted by organs on a cellular level as blood passes through tissue, and the values generally correlate inversely with rSO_2 values. Using these different measurements, NIRS devices can monitor and record data related to tissue perfusion, oxygenation, and metabolic status of various organs.

Neonates are naturally an ideal population to monitor with NIRS technology because of their small size. This is both because their organs are located close to the skin surface where NIRS light can easily penetrate and because as they are so small with fragile blood vessels, traditional invasive methods used to monitor oxygenation balance status (ie, mixed venous oxygen saturation) are impractical and seldom used.[34]

As physicians taking care of pediatric patient populations became more familiar with NIRS and more devices became commercially available (**Table 1**), they realized that the noninvasive nature and ability for continuous monitoring related to this technology was ideal in caring for critical infants. Gradually, additional NIRS monitoring of anatomic sites such as over the kidney to monitor renal rSO_2 ($RrSO_2$) and over the abdomen to monitor splanchnic rSO_2 ($SrSO_2$) were evaluated for utility and then incorporated into clinical care where deemed appropriate. Monitoring of cerebral rSO2 ($CrSO_2$), $RrSO_2$, and $SrSO_2$ have all demonstrated potential clinical usefulness.[35] NIRS is increasingly used as standard of care in certain acute care settings, such as when caring for infants with congenital cardiac disorders, because the hemodynamic status of these patients can change rapidly.[36]

Decisions about RBC transfusion all relate to oxygen carrying capacity of blood, oxygen delivery to organs, and oxygen tissue demands of organ systems. When rSO_2 values decrease, this represents either an increase in oxygen extraction by organ tissue or a decrease in oxygen delivery to tissue because of either a lower oxygen carrying capacity of blood or secondary to poor tissue perfusion.[37] NIRS devices can

Table 1
Commercially available near-infrared spectroscopy devices commonly available for potential neonatal intensive care unit monitoring

Name	Manufacturer	Manufacturer Location	Wavelengths of Light Utilized (nm)
FORE-SIGHT	Edwards Life Sciences	USA	690/730/770/810/870
INVOS	Medtronic	USA	730/810
NIRO-200 NX	Hamamatsu	Japan	735/810/850
EQUANOX	Nonin Medical	USA	730/760/810/880
Oxiplex TS	ISS	USA	690/830
Portalite mini[a]	Artinis	Netherlands	760/850
Root – 03	Masimo	USA	730/760/805/880
SenSmart	Nonin Medical	USA	730/760/810/870

[a] For research purposes only.

monitor rSO_2 and FTOE, both which highly relate to end-organ oxygen balance. Therefore, it is logical that neonatologists caring for critically ill infants, a population that receives so many transfusions and who can most benefit from noninvasive technologies, have most frequently studied how best to incorporate NIRS into RBC management.[38] NIRS has been evaluated in infants for its ability to monitor the effect that transfusion has on oxygen balance pretransfusion versus posttransfusion, to observe for anemia, and to determine when a transfusion may be best indicated.

Using Near-Infrared Spectroscopy to Understand the Effects of Red Blood Cell Transfusion on Tissue Oxygenation

To date, most pediatric researchers who have focused on the use of NIRS in context of transfusion have done so by monitoring subjects undergoing RBC transfusion and reporting changes in rSO_2 observed, often at more than one anatomic site. This has been done in an attempt to better understand the physiologic effects of RBC transfusion in the neonate. Although the brain was the earliest and most well-studied target organ in context of neonatal RBC transfusion, increasingly other anatomic sites are being used in order to have a better overall picture of distribution of blood flow and rSO_2 changes that occur in different organs under anemic conditions. Different organ NIRS monitoring is done likely in an attempt to find the most ideal potential transfusion trigger.[39]

Monitoring nonmajor organ peripheral sites, such as peripheral muscle rSO_2, has been studied in infants but is currently not commonly used in NICU clinical practice and as such is not discussed in any detail in this review.[40] **Table 2** lists many of the

Table 2
Device used and anatomic location monitored for neonatal red blood cell transfusion observational near-infrared spectroscopy studies evaluating pretransfusion and posttransfusion regional tissue oxygen saturation levels

First Author, Year of Publication	NIRS Device Used	Brain Monitoring	Abdomen Monitoring	Kidney Monitoring
Dani et al,[41] 2002	NIRO	X		
Bailey et al,[43] 2010	INVOS	X	X	
Dani et al,[42] 2010	INVOS	X	X	X
Van Hofton et al,[44] 2010	INVOS	X		
Koyano et al,[50] 2013	TRS-10	X		
Seidel et al,[45] 2013	INVOS	X		X
Mintzer et al,[48] 2014	INVOS	X	X	X
Sandal et al,[45] 2014	INVOS	X	X	
White et al,[59] 2015	FORE-SIGHT		X	
Banerjee et al,[52] 2016	NIRO	X		
Banerjee et al,[56] 2016	NIRO		X	
Li et al,[46] 2017	FORE-SIGHT	X	X	
Miller et al,[60] 2017	INVOS		X	
Weaver et al,[58] 2018	INVOS		X	
Aktas et al,[51] 2019	Sensmart	X	X	X
Jain et al,[53] 2019	INVOS	X		
Balegar et al,[63] 2022	FORE-SIGHT	X	X	
Kalteren et al,[55] 2022	INVOS		X	
Smith et al,[49] 2022	INVOS	X	X	

observational studies that have taken place during the past 2 decades, indicating which NIRS device was used and which major-organ anatomic site(s) were evaluated. Of note, transfusing 15 mL/kg of packed red blood cells (PRBC) during a 4-hour time period seems to be the norm throughout studies.

Cerebral Regional Tissue Oxygen Saturation

This NIRS parameter is the rSO_2 value that has been studied the longest, including in transfusion research. Most studies evaluating $CrSO_2$ have shown an increase that ensues in response to RBC transfusion. Sometimes the increase is short-lived, sometimes it lasts longer but rarely does $CrSO_2$ not change posttransfusion.

Early on, Dani and colleagues carried out an observational pilot study in a small group of preterm neonates who were being transfused during the first month of life and determined that there was a significant increase in $CrSO_2$ of more than 10% points immediately after the transfusion completed.[41] However, they did not monitor long enough to see if this change was sustained. Years later they published another study using a different commercially available NIRS instrument but in a similar study design and with a similar population and again found roughly the same significant short-term increase in $CrSO_2$, from about 65% to 79%.[42] This same year other researchers were reporting similar results using the same equipment but this time with cohorts of roughly 30 patients and with a longer monitoring period of up to 24 hours after transfusion and demonstrated that the increase in $CrSO_2$ was not just immediate but perhaps more sustained.[43,44] Seidel and colleagues then studied an even larger group of preterm neonates with similar technique and found that the increase in $CrSO_2$ observed posttransfusion was significantly larger in patients that started off with the lowest pretransfusion $CrSO_2$ values to begin with.[45] Meaning, RBC transfusion had a greater influence on those patients in whom oxygen carrying capacity was already more compromised, and different researchers found this too.[46] Other small studies during the past decade have continued to demonstrate a substantial increase in $CrSO_2$ after RBC transfusion.[47–49] But, rarely, researchers have found smaller changes or no change at all in $CrSO_2$ posttransfusion.[50–53]

Splanchnic Regional Tissue Oxygen Saturation

Applying NIRS to measure $SrSO_2$ during RBC transfusion is increasingly being considered and evaluated. This is likely because in an anemic state, blood vessel regulatory mechanisms will often prioritize cerebral perfusion and oxygenation at the expense of blood supply to less vital organs, including the gastrointestinal tract.[54] Therefore, theoretically, by monitoring $SrSO_2$, clinicians could see more significant change resulting from transfusion than with $CrSO_2$, or gain more insight into the transfusion needs of their patients.

Bailey and colleagues observed a larger change in $SrSO_2$ compared with $CrSO_2$ when studying approximately 30 preterm subjects during transfusion, noting values going on average from about 40% to 50% immediately after.[43] However, the $SrSO_2$ values did tend to trend down again by 12 hours after transfusion completion. The same year Dani and colleagues reported in a very similar study an even larger increase in mean $SrSO_2$ going from the mid 50% range to the mid 70% saturation level.[42] Later, 2 other NIRS research groups demonstrated that RBC transfusion resulted in a fairly large increase of approximately 15% to 20% points, with average $SrSO_2$ values ranging in the 40% to 50% range pretransfusion and 60% range posttransfusion.[47,48] Very recently, Kalteren and colleagues studied more than 50 transfusions occurring in preterm neonates and found at 24 hours, the $SrSO_2$ values had increased from a mean of about 50% to 60%.[55]

Some recent studies have observed changes in $SrSO_2$ in NICU patients getting transfusion and have evaluated the data based on age or degree of anemia. Banerjee and colleagues evaluated $SrSO_2$ by placing preterm subjects into 3 different cohorts based on day of life at time of transfusion and found that subjects in all age categories experienced an increase on average from the 40% range to the mid 50% range, independent of age.[56] Li and colleagues reported an increase of about 10% to 15% in $SrSO_2$ when studying both a group of moderately and a group of severely anemic preterm infants.[46] However, in contrast to most previous studies, they noted higher baseline $SrSO_2$ values on average, with values increasing from the middle 70% range to middle 80% range after RBC transfusion. These researchers also noted, as have others, more fluctuation and variability in $SrSO_2$ compared with a steadier signal found with $CrSO_2$.[57] Aktas and colleagues noticed a large increase of about 15% points in $SrSO_2$ following transfusion in very anemic patients (<8 g/dL), from the low 60% range to low/mid 70% range but noted hardly any increase in $SrSO_2$ in the other neonates being transfused and monitored.[51] One group very recently saw an increase of 20% in $SrSO_2$ at 24 hours when transfusing preterm patients without a patent ductus arteriosus (PDA), but saw no change at all, and much lower baseline $SrSO_2$ values, when monitoring transfusions of patients who had significant PDAs.[49] This demonstrates how other factors other than just anemia can affect rSO_2 levels. The largest increase in $SrSO_2$ observed to date was from a study of about 30 preterm subjects with Hgb values lesser than 8 g/dL in which there was a significant increase in $SrSO_2$ following transfusion from the low 40% range to the high 70% range.[58]

As with $CrSO_2$, a few researchers have not found much of a change in $SrSO_2$ with transfusion. When White and colleagues investigated RBC transfusion and $SrSO_2$ change, at up to 36 hours, these researchers did not see a significant change. However, when evaluating NIRS for up to 48 hours, they then did see a small change in $SrSO_2$ that was statistically significant, with $SrSO_2$ going on average from the mid/high 60% to just about 70%.[59] Another group did not find hardly any increase, and then after transfusion, the $SrSO_2$ actually went down immediately after.[60] One last group recently also found no significant change in abdominal NIRS values but their sensor placement was over the liver and they were evaluating a group of preterm subjects being transfused using a liberal strategy.[61] This demonstrates some of the variability that can exist when attempting abdominal NIRS monitoring.

Renal Regional Tissue Oxygen Saturation

Renal tissue oxygenation is the least-studied NIRS parameters in relation to RBC transfusion. However, there are studies that have evaluated the changes that occur in $RrSO_2$ with transfusion, usually while also evaluating other parameters. The earliest study in infants to evaluate for this demonstrated that RBC transfusion had about the same effect on $RrSO_2$ as it did on $CrSO_2$ with a more than 10% point increase immediately after transfusion.[42] These authors also studied the renal arterial blood velocity and did not observe a difference, meaning that the increase in $RrSO_2$ was likely due to increased oxygen carrying capacity of blood rather than an increase in perfusion. Other researchers also found at least the same increase in $RrSO_2$ in a group of more than 70 preterm subjects undergoing transfusion but did not see a more significant increase in those who began with lower tissue oxygenation levels.[45] Mintzer and colleagues found the largest change in tissue oxygen saturation that occurred posttransfusion was in $RrSO_2$ values and that it was an almost 20% increase, compared with 10% for $CrSO_2$.[48] Finally, and most recently, Aktas and colleagues found only a small increase in $RrSO_2$ of just 2% after RBC transfusion using a newer NIRS device, although it was statistically significant.[51] All of these studies only evaluated patients in the immediate posttransfusion period.

In summary, $RrSO_2$ does seem to increase consistently with RBC transfusion, and in general, it may increase as much, if not more, than $CrSO_2$. One reason for this, again, could be that although the kidney vessels do try to maintain consistent blood flow, the cerebral vasculature has even more enhanced autoregulatory mechanisms to permit adequate perfusion during anemic states.

Splanchnic-Cerebral Oxygenation Ratio

Measuring 2 NIRS values simultaneously and in conjunction, as a ratio, has been thought to be potentially helpful in determining physiologic changes that may be occurring in the body. The main ratio that has been used in this manner in neonatal medicine is the splanchnic-cerebral oxygenation ratio (SCOR) that compares $SrSO_2$ in relation to $CrSO_2$: $SCOR = SrSO_2/CrSO_2$. In a very anemic state, it is likely possible that gastrointestinal blood flow would decrease in order to preserve blood flow and perfusion to the brain, and the SCOR would subsequently decrease. Therefore, researchers have looked to see if there is a change in this ratio that occurs after RBC transfusion.

One of the first studies to report on SCOR in this manner evaluated a group of symptomatic preterm infants who were administered RBC transfusion.[62] After transfusion, the investigators looked to see which subjects clinically improved. As a group of total subjects, the mean SCOR increased from baseline after transfusion. When they broke down the evaluation based on improvement parameters, they found that those subjects who improved on average had a significant increase in their SCOR from 0.61 to 0.76 and those that did not improve had only an increase from 0.75 to 0.81. Another similar study was reported 2 years later by Sandal and colleagues and validated these results. This research group reported a mean SCOR of 0.64 before transfusion in symptomatic subjects that increased to 0.81 after transfusion with RBCs.[47]

The most recent study looking at SCOR changes during transfusion actually showed a downward trend, instead of upward, after transfusion. In that article by Balegar and colleagues, they showed the SCOR go from about 1.17 to approximately 1.11 after transfusion, and these values were sustained for 24 hours after the RBC transfusion. In this case, the mean $SrSO_2$ stayed consistent at 83% and the $CrSO_2$ increased from about 72% to 74%. One difference in this study from the others is that different NIRS monitors were used, although the same specific anatomic locations were studied.[63]

Fractional Tissue Oxygen Extraction

FTOE is another NIRS parameter that has been well studied in neonatal transfusion medicine. However, unlike the other NIRS values, FTOE is a derived value because it is calculated based on the rSO_2 value and the SaO_2 value observed simultaneously. As previously mentioned, FTOE is inversely correlated to rSO_2 as oxygen saturation values usually are between 90% and 95% in preterm patients. Because most of the reports on FTOE are from the same studies as discussed in the other sections, we will only briefly discuss FTOE here.

Dani and colleagues noted a reduction in cerebral, splanchnic, and renal FTOE following RBC transfusion in symptomatic preterm patients.[42] In another observational study of more than 30 preterm subject, van Hoften and colleagues found that cerebral FTOE decreased also significantly after transfusion.[44] As a final example, when Mintzer and colleagues evaluated multiple-organ FTOE changes, they found that there was a decrease in cerebral, renal, and splanchnic tissue FTOE of 27%,

30%, and 9%, respectively, that resulted from transfusion in a preterm population of patients in the NICU.[48]

THE CORRELATION OF NEAR-INFRARED SPECTROSCOPY VALUES WITH HEMOGLOBIN OR HEMATOCRIT LEVELS

Although there have been many studies looking at changes in various NIRS parameters as a result of transfusion, only a handful have reported on the correlation found, if any, between rSO_2 and Hgb levels. The studies all have relatively small sample sizes, and the conclusions are mixed.

Bailey and colleagues did not find any significant correlation between both pretransfusion Hgb levels and $CrSO_2$ measurements, as well as posttransfusion Hgb levels and $CrSO_2$ measurements.[43] In addition, $SrSO_2$ was evaluated in the same context, and again, no significant correlation between Hgb and $SrSO_2$ was found, either in the pretransfusion or in the posttransfusion state. In a later study with twice as many monitored transfusions, the authors also concluded that there was not a correlation found between Hgb and NIRS parameters.[45]

In contrast, Andersen and colleagues demonstrated a significant correlation between pretransfusion Hgb and $CrSO_2$ in 2 dozen preterm infants being monitored with NIRS during RBC transfusion.[64] Another group also found a correlation between $CrSO_2$ and Hgb and determined that $CrSO_2$ may be at risk when Hgb values decrease to less than 9.5 g/dL.[44] Finally, Mintzer and colleagues reported a mixed picture. They found that cerebral FTOE and renal FTOE inversely correlated with HCT but that there was no correlation between splanchnic FTOE and HCT.[65]

The answer to the correlation question remains unclear, and further studies are required to address this. If there was an obvious and direct correlation, then perhaps NIRS would not add further value as a transfusion trigger because it would simply be providing similar information that obtaining a Hgb or HCT could determine. Alternatively, maybe NIRS could be used in a similar way as a transcutaneous CO_2 detector is used in conjunction with obtaining intermittent blood gas values for intubated patients.[66] However, because a correlation remains unknown, this further demonstrates that NIRS may still hold value as a physiologic indicator of transfusion need, and possibly be better than Hgb in this regard.

NEAR-INFRARED SPECTROSCOPY TO GUIDE RED BLOOD CELL TRANSFUSION IN NEONATES

There are few studies directly evaluating the use of NIRS to guide neonatal RBC transfusion, and only one is a prospective randomized study. It is an investigation of preterm infants comparing NIRS-guided transfusion management versus traditional methods.[67] In this study by Wardle and colleagues, these investigators monitored peripheral muscle rSO_2 with NIRS and used either an FTOE greater than 0.47 or clinical concern by the physician to trigger transfusion in the study group. In the control group, subjects were transfused based on Hgb level and oxygen requirement, or if the patient was demonstrating significant clinical signs of anemia based on preset criteria. Although there were less total transfusions administered in the NIRS group, the difference was not statistically significant, and the average number of transfusions given to each individual subject did not differ. However, a major limitation of this study was that more transfusions in the NIRS group took place because of clinician concern than because of an elevated FTOE. This could possibly mean that the medical team did not trust NIRS as a technology for this use, or perhaps the researchers set the FTOE transfusion trigger too high. Either way, this study may not be a completely objective analysis of the utilization of NIRS for this purpose. This same research team also evaluated in a different observational study the FTOE values of preterm subjects divided into 3 groups: asymptomatic infants given a transfusion, symptomatic infants given transfusion, and an asymptomatic control group.[68] They found that the mean pretransfusion FTOE was 0.43 in the symptomatic transfused group, significantly higher than 0.33 and 0.35 in the other 2 groups and concluded that FTOE could be a useful transfusion marker. It is important to note that both of these studies used peripheral muscle NIRS monitoring, which as noted early, does not seem to be commonly recommended for routine NICU clinical use at this time.[40]

Other studies that have discussed the use of NIRS to determine RBC transfusion need in infants have done so mainly by retrospectively analyzing data they obtained in an observational manner and breaking subjects down into groups based on whether researchers determined that the patient improved or not after a transfusion. For example, Bailey and colleagues using a post hoc analysis and receiver operator curve demonstrated that an SCOR of less than 0.73 could be used to help identify preterm neonates who will benefit from RBC transfusion.[62] Later, Seidel and colleagues recommended that a $CrSO_2$ of less than 55% could indicate that an infant would benefit from transfusion.[45] However, the methodology used to come up with these conclusions and others has potential flaws and requires larger prospective studies evaluating these parameters for validation.

The most recent study related to whether NIRS could aid in NICU RBC transfusion management comes from a substudy of the Transfusion of Prematures trial in which investigators were comparing a low Hgb versus higher Hgb transfusion threshold criteria in infants with ELBW.[8] Chock and colleagues investigated if there was any difference in $CrSO_2$ or $SrSO_2$ during the first week of life in these same subjects.[69] They found that infants who had a greater degree of anemia, those in the low-Hgb threshold group requiring 2 or more transfusions, also had the lowest $CrSO_2$ values and highest cerebral FTOE values. Although this study does not answer the question of how NIRS could be exactly used in this capacity, it does suggest how it might be used as an adjunctive tool.

LIMITATIONS

Although the ability of NIRS to help successfully guide RBC transfusion practice in neonates holds great promise, there are limitations with the studies examining this along with limitations of the technology itself. Both may have hampered its widespread adoption for this use indication. There are also increased hospital costs associated with NIRS equipment purchases and maintenance, along with more required training of staff, which pose additional barriers.[70]

In regards to neonatal NIRS transfusion study limitations, there are several.[71] First, most NIRS transfusion studies are small, single-center observational trials, determining tissue oxygenation changes that occur with RBC transfusion, rather than evaluating NIRS as a tool to determine transfusion triggers in a prospective manner. There is also a high degree of heterogenicity among these studies, with different NIRS devices being used for measurements, different anatomic locations evaluated, and different RBC transfusion triggers and practices used. In addition, there is not consistency in populations studied, with varying degrees of comorbidities, and monitoring taking place during various periods. Comorbid conditions that exist within these neonatal study subjects, such as PDA or infection, for example, can alter hemodynamics both on a macrovascular and microvascular level, thus leading to differences in rSO_2 not related to an anemic state.[72,73] The studies that examined NIRS derived cutoff values that may warrant RBC transfusion had different recommendations based on varying techniques. Finally, most studies did not consistently evaluate subjects who did not receive transfusion to determine if there is any clinical detriment and rSO_2 correlation.

There are also some limitations of NIRS as a technology as it is currently in use. First, there is a lack of standardization in equipment that is used clinically. Different NIRS device manufacturers can use somewhat different wavelengths of light, at varying depths of penetration, and have their own proprietary algorithms that calculate an rSO_2 value.[74] This often leads to a common question related to NIRS: should it be used only as a trend monitor or as a device that can provide absolute values that can trigger some action?[75] One possible work-around of this issue can be the use of rSO_2 ratio values (ie, SCOR), as if one is using 2 rSO_2 trends and monitoring how they are changing in context of each other, and this could nullify the issue. This point highlights also that different anatomic sites with different NIRS parameters (ie, $CrSO_2$, $RrSO_2$, and $SrSO_2$) are monitored, often without consistency. Even when choosing to measure rSO_2 in the same anatomic site, there are different locations that the sensors can be placed. For example, when monitoring $SrSO_2$, sensors are commonly placed midline and below the umbilicus but others may place sensors over other areas on the abdomen, leading to varying rSO_2 value measurements.[76] All of this variation in practice discussed, further contributes to the difficulty in making any conclusive recommendations about NIRS clinical use for transfusion decision-making.

NEXT STEPS

Further clinical evidence is required before NIRS monitoring can routinely be incorporated as a standard care practice into the guidance of neonatal RBC transfusion therapy. Based on all of the previous research, it seems reasonable that NIRS can be used to monitor rSO_2 changes that occur in various organs. What exactly those changes mean and how long these changes last for is still in question. If additional, larger observational research is to be conducted, it should improve on previous study by monitoring subjects for longer periods with NIRS along with the clinical outcomes after transfusion.

However, the next phase of clinical studies evaluating the use of NIRS in context of RBC transfusion should ideally be prospective randomized control trials, either evaluating the use of NIRS as a stand-alone transfusion marker, or as part of a transfusion decision-making algorithm that may also incorporate Hgb levels and/or clinical signs of anemia. These studies would likely be multicentered and use a uniform group of preterm neonatal subjects with clear inclusion and exclusion criteria in order to eliminate as many confounding factors as possible. The research protocols should also use strict transfusion criteria in the control group and make sure that for both groups, RBC storage times and administration processes are the same. If these studies show promise with a select group of preterm subjects, then further research could be expanded more broadly to include other infants cared for in an NICU setting.

Neonatologists may also consider using NIRS equipment that is currently available in many NICUS to monitor select patients under their care. NIRS could help gather additional physiologic information that may be helpful when making transfusion decisions in cases that are unclear based on current standard guidelines. If a patient is a borderline case, NIRS data could help influence an RBC transfusion decision by either offering evidence that tissue oxygenation and perfusion is adequate, or suggesting the contrary.

SUMMARY

In conclusion, NIRS seems as a well-studied method to monitor rSO_2 in infants that has promising potential for use in the management of RBC transfusion. Currently, there is a lack of evidence to support recommending the use of NIRS-derived values to determine specific transfusion needs of patients during neonatal intensive care. However, clinicians could expand their use of this technology when caring for neonates in order to gather more data on the physiologic status of their patients. Further studies are needed, especially larger prospective randomized controlled trials, before widespread implementation of NIRS into transfusion management should occur. In addition, neonatal care teams will need to think about how best to implement this equipment into their overall transfusion strategies, such as a single marker of transfusion need, or as just one component of an RBC transfusion protocol. Neonatology as a field is clearly moving toward a more individualized patient approach to care. Using NIRS as a tool to indicate when a specific patient would benefit from RBC transfusion could be one of the next steps along this path.

Best Practices Box

What is the Current Practice?

Currently, Hgb and HCT are used as the primary markers of red blood cell transfusion need during neonatal intensive care, and restrictive transfusion guidelines using lower value thresholds are thought to be equivalent to liberal guidelines that lead to more transfusions.

What changes in current practice are likely to improve outcomes?

The use of more specific markers of red blood cell transfusion need could limit the number of unnecessary transfusions that are administered in a neonatal population. Ultimately, this could perhaps reduce resources used in the care of preterm infants and potentially improve both short-term and long-term outcomes in this vulnerable patient population.

Major Recommendations

- NIRS should be studied in large prospective randomized controlled trials in order to determine if this technology could be helpful in guiding red blood cell transfusion practice in neonatal intensive care.
- NIRS can be monitored in neonatal patients to gather additional physiologic information that could help influence neonatal clinicians when making transfusion decisions in situations that are unclear based on using Hgb or HCT values alone.

DISCLOSURE

Dr S.M. Bailey is a member of the Medtronic speaker bureau. Dr P.V. Mally has nothing to disclose.

REFERENCES

1. Zerra PE, Josephson CD. Transfusion in neonatal patients: review of evidence-based guidelines. Clin Lab Med 2021;41(1):15–34.
2. Villeneuve A, Arsenault V, Lacroix J, et al. Neonatal red blood cell transfusion. Vox Sang 2021;116(4):366–78.
3. Keir AK, Yang J, Harrison A, et al, Canadian Neonatal Network. Temporal changes in blood product usage in preterm neonates born at less than 30 weeks' gestation in Canada. Transfusion 2015;55(6):1340–6.

4. Valieva OA, Strandjord TP, Mayock DE, et al. Effects of transfusions in extremely low birth weight infants: a retrospective study. J Pediatr 2009;155(3):331–7.
5. Collard KJ. Transfusion related morbidity in premature babies: possible mechanisms and implications for practice. World J Clin Pediatr 2014;3(3):19–29.
6. Bell EF. Red cell transfusion thresholds for preterm infants: Finally, some answers. Arch Dis Child Fetal Neonatal Ed 2022;107(2):126–30.
7. Franz AR, Engel C, Bassler D, et al. Effects of liberal vs restrictive transfusion thresholds on survival and neurocognitive outcomes in extremely low-birth-weight infants: the ETTNO randomized clinical trial. JAMA 2020;324(6):560–70.
8. Kirpalani H, Bell EF, Hintz SR, et al. Higher or lower hemoglobin transfusion thresholds for preterm infants. N Engl J Med 2020;383(27):2639–51.
9. Wang YC, Chan OW, Chiang MC, et al. Red blood cell transfusion and clinical outcomes in extremely low birth weight preterm infants. Pediatr Neonatol 2017; 58(3):216–22.
10. Mally P, Golombek SG, Mishra R, et al. Association of necrotizing enterocolitis with elective packed red blood cell transfusions in stable, growing, premature neonates. Am J Perinatol 2006;23(8):451–8.
11. Slidsborg C, Jensen A, Forman JL, et al. Neonatal risk factors for treatment-demanding retinopathy of prematurity: a Danish National Study. Ophthalmology 2016;23:796–803.
12. Baer VL, Lambert DK, Henry E, et al. Red blood cell transfusion of preterm neonates with a Grade 1 intraventricular hemorrhage is associated with extension to a Grade 3 or 4 hemorrhage. Transfusion 2011;51:1933–9.
13. Vlaar AP. Transfusion-related acute lung injury: current understanding and preventive strategies. Transfus Clin Biol 2012;19(3):117–24.
14. Wang JK, Klein HG. Red blood cell transfusion in the treatment and management of anaemia: the search for the elusive transfusion trigger. Vox Sang 2010; 98(1):2–11.
15. Andersen CC, Keir AK, Kirpalani HM, et al. Anaemia in the premature infant and red blood cell transfusion: new approaches to an age-old problem. Curr Treat Options Peds 2015;1:191–201.
16. Tsai AG, Hofmann A, Cabrales P, et al. Perfusion vs. oxygen delivery in transfusion with "fresh" and "old" red blood cells: the experimental evidence. Transfus Apher Sci 2010;43(1):69–78.
17. Kasat K, Hendricks-Muñoz KD, Mally PV. Neonatal red blood cell transfusions: searching for better guidelines. Blood Transfus 2011;9(1):86–94.
18. Kanmaz HG, Sarikabadayi YU, Canpolat E, et al. Effects of red cell transfusion on cardiac output and perfusion index in preterm infants. Early Hum Dev 2013;89(9): 683–6.
19. Czempik PF, Gierczak D, Wilczek D, et al. The impact of red blood cell transfusion on blood lactate in non-bleeding critically ill patients-A retrospective cohort study. J Clin Med 2022;11(4):1037.
20. Ibonia KT, Bada HS, Westgate PM, et al. Blood transfusions in preterm infants: changes on perfusion index and intermittent hypoxemia. Transfusion 2018; 58(11):2538–44.
21. Pavlek LR, Mueller C, Jebbia MR, et al. Near-infrared spectroscopy in extremely preterm infants. Front Pediatr 2021;8:624113.
22. Whyte R, Kirpalani H. Low versus high haemoglobin concentration threshold for blood transfusion for preventing morbidity and mortality in very low birth weight infants. Cochrane Database Syst Rev 2011;11:CD000512.

23. Red Blood cell transfusions in newborn infants: revised guidelines. Paediatr Child Health 2002;7:553–66.

24. Roseff SD, Luban N, Manno CS. Guidelines for assessing appropriateness of pediatric transfusion. Transfusion 2002;42:1398–413.

25. Nakhla D, Kushnir A, Ahmed R, et al. Reticulocyte count: the forgotten factor in transfusion decisions for extremely low birth weight infants. Am J Perinatol 2021. https://doi.org/10.1055/a-1653-4585.

26. Howarth C, Banerjee J, Aladangady N. Red blood cell transfusion in preterm infants: current evidence and controversies. Neonatology 2018;114(1):7–16.

27. Guillén U, Cummings JJ, Bell EF, et al. International survey of transfusion practices for extremely premature infants. Semin Perinatol 2012;36(4):244–7.

28. Patel RM, Hendrickson JE, Nellis ME, et al. Variation in neonatal transfusion practice. J Pediatr 2021;235:92–9.e4.

29. Meyer MP, O'Connor KL, Meyer JH. Thresholds for blood transfusion in extremely preterm infants: a review of the latest evidence from two large clinical trials. Front Pediatr 2022;10:957585.

30. Franchini M, Marano G, Mengoli C, et al. Red blood cell transfusion policy: a critical literature review. Blood Transfus 2017;15(4):307–31.

31. Scrivens A, Reibel NJ, Heeger L, et al. Survey of transfusion practices in preterm infants in Europe. Arch Dis Child Fetal Neonatal Ed 2023. fetalneonatal-2022-324619.

32. Wolfberg AJ, du Plessis AJ. Near infrared spectroscopy in the fetus and neonata. Clin Perinatol 2006;33(3):707–28.

33. Marin T, Moore J. Understanding near-infrared spectroscopy. Adv Neonatal Care 2011;11(6):382–8.

34. Ghanayem NS, Wernovsky G, Hoffman GM. Near-infrared spectroscopy as a hemodynamic monitor in critical illness. Pediatr Crit Care Med 2011;12(4 Suppl): S27–32.

35. Evans KM, Rubarth LB. Investigating the role of near-infrared spectroscopy in neonatal medicine. Neonatal Netw 2017;36(4):189–95.

36. Zaleski KL, Kussman BD. Near-infrared spectroscopy in pediatric congenital heart disease. J Cardiothorac Vasc Anesth 2020;34(2):489–500.

37. Saroha V, Josephson CD, Patel RM. Epidemiology of necrotizing enterocolitis: new considerations regarding the influence of red blood cell transfusions and anemia. Clin Perinatol 2019;46(1):101–17.

38. Crispin P, Forwood K. Near infrared spectroscopy in anemia detection and management: a systematic review. Transfus Med Rev 2021;35(1):22–8.

39. Banerjee J, Aladangady N. Biomarkers to decide red blood cell transfusion in newborn infants. Transfusion 2014;54(10):2574–82.

40. Höller N, Urlesberger B, Mileder L, et al. Peripheral muscle near-infrared spectroscopy in neonates: ready for clinical use? A systematic qualitative review of the literature. Neonatology 2015;108(4):233–45.

41. Dani C, Pezzati M, Martelli E, et al. Acta Paediatr 2002;91(9):938–41.

42. Dani C, Pratesi S, Fontanelli G, et al. Blood transfusions increase cerebral, splanchnic,and renal oxygenation in anemic preterm infants. Transfusion 2010; 50(6):1220–6.

43. Bailey SM, Hendricks-Muñoz KD, Wells JT, et al. Packed red blood cell transfusion increases regional cerebral and splanchnic tissue oxygen saturation in anemic symptomatic preterm infants. Am J Perinatol 2010;27(6):445–53.

44. van Hoften JC, Verhagen EA, Keating P, et al. Cerebral tissue oxygen saturation and extraction in preterm infants before and after blood transfusion. Arch Dis Child Fetal Neonatal Ed 2010;95(5):F352–8.
45. Seidel D, Bläser A, Gebauer C, et al. Changes in regional tissue oxygenation saturation and desaturations after red blood cell transfusion in preterm infants. J Perinatol 2013;33(4):282–7.
46. Li L, Wu R, Kog X, et al. Effect of anemia and blood transfusion on tissue oxygen saturation and blood pressure in very preterm infants. Int J Clin Exp Med 2017; 10:2974–9.
47. Sandal G, Oguz SS, Erdeve O, et al. Assessment of red blood cell transfusion and transfusion duration on cerebral and mesenteric oxygenation using near-infrared spectroscopy in preterm infants with symptomatic anemia. Transfusion 2014;54(4):1100–5.
48. Mintzer JP, Parvez B, Chelala M, et al. Monitoring regional tissue oxygen extraction in neonates <1250 g helps identify transfusion thresholds independent of hematocrit. J Neonatal Perinat Med 2014;7(2):89–100.
49. Smith A, Armstrong S, Dempsey E, et al. The impact of a PDA on tissue oxygenation and haemodynamics following a blood transfusion in preterm infants. Pediatr Res 2022;93(5):1314–20.
50. Koyano K, Kusaka T, Nakamura S, et al. The effect of blood transfusion on cerebral hemodynamics in preterm infants. Transfusion 2013;53(7):1459–67.
51. Aktas S, Ergenekon E, Ozcan E, et al. Effects of blood transfusion on regional tissue oxygenation in preterm newborns are dependent on the degree of anaemia. J Paediatr Child Health 2019;55(10):1209–13.
52. Banerjee J, Leung TS, Aladangady N. Cerebral blood flow and oximetry response to blood transfusion in relation to chronological age in preterm infants. Early Hum Dev 2016;97:1–8.
53. Jain D, D'Ugard C, Bancalari E, et al. Cerebral oxygenation in preterm infants receiving transfusion. Pediatr Res 2019;85(6):786–9. https://doi.org/10.1038/s41390-018-0266-7.
54. Dantsker DR. The gastrointestinal tract: the canary of the body? JAMA 1993;270: 1247–8.
55. Kalteren WS, Bos AF, Bergman KA, et al. The short-term effects of RBC transfusions on intestinal isnjury in preterm infants. Pediatr Res 2022;1–7. https://doi.org/10.1038/s41390-022-01961-9.
56. Banerjee J, Leung TS, Aladangady N. Blood transfusion in preterm infants improves intestinal tissue oxygenation without alteration in blood flow. Vox Sang 2016;111(4):399–408.
57. Bailey SM, Hendricks-Muñoz KD, Mally PV. Variability in splanchnic tissue oxygenation during preterm red blood cell transfusion given for symptomatic anaemia may reveal a potential mechanism of transfusion-related acute gut injury. Blood Transfus 2015;13(3):429–34.
58. Weaver B, Guerreso K, Conner EA, et al. Hemodynamics and perfusion in premature infants during transfusion. AACN Adv Crit Care 2018;29(2):126–37. Summer.
59. White L, Said M, Rais-Bahrami K. Monitoring mesenteric tissue oxygenation with near-infrared spectroscopy during packed red blood cell transfusion in preterm infants. J Neonatal Perinat Med 2015;8(2):157–63.
60. Miller HD, Penoyer DA, Baumann K, et al. Assessment of mesenteric tissue saturation, oxygen saturation, and heart rate pre- and post-blood transfusion in very low-birth-weight infants using abdominal site near-infrared spectroscopy. Adv Neonatal Care 2017;17(5):E3–9.

61. Jani P, Lowe K, Hinder M, et al. Changes to hepatic tissue oxygenation, abdominal perfusion and its association with enteral feeding with liberal transfusion threshold in anaemic preterm infants: a prospective cohort study. Vox Sang 2020;115(8):712–21.
62. Bailey SM, Hendricks-Muñoz KD, Mally P. Splanchnic-cerebral oxygenation ratio as a marker of preterm infant blood transfusion needs. Transfusion 2012;52(2): 252–60.
63. Balegar VKK, Jayawardhana M, de Chazal P, et al. Splanchnic-cerebral oxygenation ratio associated with packed red blood cell transfusion in preterm infants. Transfus Med 2022;32(6):475–83.
64. Andersen CC, Karayil SM, Hodyl NA, et al. Early red cell transfusion favourably alters cerebral oxygen extraction in very preterm newborns. Arch Dis Child Fetal Neonatal Ed 2015;100(5):F433–5.
65. Mintzer JP, Parvez B, La Gamma EF. Regional tissue oxygen extraction and severity of anemia in very low birth weight neonates: a pilot NIRS analysis. Am J Perinatol 2018;35(14):1411–8.
66. Hochwald O, Borenstein-Levin L, Dinur G, et al. Continuous noninvasive carbon dioxide monitoring in neonates: from theory to standard of care. Pediatrics 2019; 144(1):e20183640.
67. Wardle SP, Garr R, Yoxall CW, et al. A pilot randomised controlled trial of peripheral fractional oxygen extraction to guide blood transfusions in preterm infants. Arch Dis Child Fetal Neonatal Ed 2002;86(1):F22–7.
68. Wardle SP, Yoxall CW, Crawley E, et al. Peripheral oxygenation and anemia in preterm babies. Pediatr Res 1998;44(1):125–31.
69. Chock VY, Smith E, Tan S, et al. Early brain and abdominal oxygenation in extremely low birth weight infants. Pediatr Res 2022;92(4):1034–41.
70. Hirsch JC, Charpie JR, Ohye RG, et al. Near infrared spectroscopy (NIRS) should not be standard of care for postoperative management. Semin Thorac Cardiovasc Surg Pediatr Card Surg Annu 2010;13(1):51–4.
71. Jani P, Balegarvirupakshappa K, Moore JE, et al. Regional oxygenation and perfusion monitoring to optimize neonatal packed red blood cell transfusion practices: a systematic review. Transfus Med Rev 2022;36(1):27–47.
72. Chock VY, Rose LA, Mante JV, et al. Near-infrared spectroscopy for detection of a significant patent ductus arteriosus. Pediatr Res 2016;80:675–80.
73. Shapiro NI, Arnold R, R Sherwin, et al. The association of near-infrared spectroscopy-derived tissue oxygenation measurements with sepsis syndromes, organ dysfunction and mortality in emergency department patients with sepsis. Crit Care 2011;15(5):R223.
74. Nagdyman N, Ewert P, Peters B, et al. Comparison of different near-infrared spectroscopic cerebral oxygenation indices with central venous and jugular venous oxygenation saturation in children. Paediatr Anaesth 2008;18(2):160–6.
75. Murkin JM, Arango M. Near-infrared spectroscopy as an index of brain and tissue oxygenation. Br J Anaesth 2009;103(Suppl 1):i3–13.
76. Goldshtrom N, Isler JR, Sahni R. Comparing liver and lower abdomen near-infrared spectroscopy in preterm infants. Early Hum Dev 2020;151:105194.

UNITED STATES POSTAL SERVICE®

Statement of Ownership, Management, and Circulation
(All Periodicals Publications Except Requester Publications)

1. Publication Title
CLINICS IN PERINATOLOGY

2. Publication Number
001 – 744

3. Filing Date
9/18/2023

4. Issue Frequency
MAR, JUN, SEP, DEC

5. Number of Issues Published Annually
4

6. Annual Subscription Price
$341.00

7. Complete Mailing Address of Known Office of Publication *(Not printer)* *(Street, city, county, state, and ZIP+4®)*
ELSEVIER INC.
230 Park Avenue, Suite 800
New York, NY 10169

Contact Person: Malathi Samayan
Telephone *(Include area code)*: 91-44-4296-4507

8. Complete Mailing Address of Headquarters or General Business Office of Publisher *(Not printer)*
ELSEVIER INC.
230 Park Avenue, Suite 800
New York, NY 10169

9. Full Names and Complete Mailing Addresses of Publisher, Editor, and Managing Editor *(Do not leave blank)*

Publisher *(Name and complete mailing address)*
DOLORES MELONI, ELSEVIER INC.
1600 JOHN F KENNEDY BLVD. SUITE 1600
PHILADELPHIA, PA 19103-2899

Editor *(Name and complete mailing address)*
KERRY HOLLAND, ELSEVIER INC.
1600 JOHN F KENNEDY BLVD. SUITE 1600
PHILADELPHIA, PA 19103-2899

Managing Editor *(Name and complete mailing address)*
PATRICK MANLEY, ELSEVIER INC.
1600 JOHN F KENNEDY BLVD. SUITE 1600
PHILADELPHIA, PA 19103-2899

10. Owner *(Do not leave blank. If the publication is owned by a corporation, give the name and address of the corporation immediately followed by the names and addresses of all stockholders owning or holding 1 percent or more of the total amount of stock. If not owned by a corporation, give the names and addresses of the individual owners. If owned by a partnership or other unincorporated firm, give its name and address as well as those of each individual owner. If the publication is published by a nonprofit organization, give its name and address.)*

Full Name	Complete Mailing Address
WHOLLY OWNED SUBSIDIARY OF REED/ELSEVIER, US HOLDINGS	1600 JOHN F KENNEDY BLVD. SUITE 1600 PHILADELPHIA, PA 19103-2899

11. Known Bondholders, Mortgagees, and Other Security Holders Owning or Holding 1 Percent or More of Total Amount of Bonds, Mortgages, or Other Securities. If none, check box ☑ None

Full Name	Complete Mailing Address
N/A	

12. Tax Status *(For completion by nonprofit organizations authorized to mail at nonprofit rates)* *(Check one)*
The purpose, function, and nonprofit status of this organization and the exempt status for federal income tax purposes:
☒ Has Not Changed During Preceding 12 Months
☐ Has Changed During Preceding 12 Months *(Publisher must submit explanation of change with this statement)*

PS Form **3526**, July 2014 *[Page 1 of 4 (see instructions page 4)]* PSN: 7530-01-000-9931 PRIVACY NOTICE: See our privacy policy on www.usps.com.

---

13. Publication Title
CLINICS IN PERINATOLOGY

14. Issue Date for Circulation Data Below
JUNE 2023

15. Extent and Nature of Circulation

			Average No. Copies Each Issue During Preceding 12 Months	No. Copies of Single Issue Published Nearest to Filing Date
a. Total Number of Copies *(Net press run)*			431	385
b. Paid Circulation *(By Mail and Outside the Mail)*	(1)	Mailed Outside-County Paid Subscriptions Stated on PS Form 3541 (Include paid distribution above nominal rate, advertiser's proof copies, and exchange copies)	346	311
	(2)	Mailed In-County Paid Subscriptions Stated on PS Form 3541 (Include paid distribution above nominal rate, advertiser's proof copies, and exchange copies)	0	0
	(3)	Paid Distribution Outside the Mails Including Sales Through Dealers and Carriers, Street Vendors, Counter Sales, and Other Paid Distribution Outside USPS®	69	58
	(4)	Paid Distribution by Other Classes of Mail Through the USPS (e.g., First-Class Mail®)	12	12
c. Total Paid Distribution *(Sum of 15b (1), (2), (3), and (4))*			427	381
d. Free or Nominal Rate Distribution *(By Mail and Outside the Mail)*	(1)	Free or Nominal Rate Outside-County Copies included on PS Form 3541	4	3
	(2)	Free or Nominal Rate In-County Copies Included on PS Form 3541	0	0
	(3)	Free or Nominal Rate Copies Mailed at Other Classes Through the USPS (e.g., First-Class Mail)	0	0
	(4)	Free or Nominal Rate Distribution Outside the Mail (Carriers or other means)	1	1
e. Total Free or Nominal Rate Distribution *(Sum of 15d (1), (2), (3) and (4))*			5	4
f. Total Distribution *(Sum of 15c and 15e)*			431	385
g. Copies not Distributed *(See Instructions to Publishers #4 (page #3))*			0	0
h. Total *(Sum of 15f and g)*			431	385
i. Percent Paid *(15c divided by 15f times 100)*			98.95%	98.96%

* If you are claiming electronic copies, go to line 16 on page 3. If you are not claiming electronic copies, skip to line 17 on page 3.

PS Form 3526, July 2014 *(Page 2 of 4)*

16. Electronic Copy Circulation

		Average No. Copies Each Issue During Preceding 12 Months	No. Copies of Single Issue Published Nearest to Filing Date
a. Paid Electronic Copies	▶		
b. Total Paid Print Copies (Line 15c) + Paid Electronic Copies (Line 16a)	▶		
c. Total Print Distribution (Line 15f) + Paid Electronic Copies (Line 16a)	▶		
d. Percent Paid (Both Print & Electronic Copies) (16b divided by 16c × 100)	▶		

☒ I certify that 50% of all my distributed copies (electronic and print) are paid above a nominal price.

17. Publication of Statement of Ownership
☒ If the publication is a general publication, publication of this statement is required. Will be printed in the DECEMBER 2023 issue of this publication. ☐ Publication not required.

18. Signature and Title of Editor, Publisher, Business Manager, or Owner

Malathi Samayan - Distribution Controller   *Malathi Samayan*

Date 9/18/2023

I certify that all information furnished on this form is true and complete. I understand that anyone who furnishes false or misleading information on this form or who omits material or information requested on the form may be subject to criminal sanctions (including fines and imprisonment) and/or civil sanctions (including civil penalties).

PS Form **3526**, July 2014 *(Page 3 of 4)* PRIVACY NOTICE: See our privacy policy on www.usps.com.

Moving?

Make sure your subscription moves with you!

To notify us of your new address, find your **Clinics Account Number** (located on your mailing label above your name), and contact customer service at:

Email: journalscustomerservice-usa@elsevier.com

800-654-2452 (subscribers in the U.S. & Canada)
314-447-8871 (subscribers outside of the U.S. & Canada)

Fax number: 314-447-8029

Elsevier Health Sciences Division
Subscription Customer Service
3251 Riverport Lane
Maryland Heights, MO 63043

*To ensure uninterrupted delivery of your subscription, please notify us at least 4 weeks in advance of move.

Printed and bound by CPI Group (UK) Ltd, Croydon, CR0 4YY

03/10/2024

01040469-0014